Lotus of a Conscious Rebirth

FRANCES MAHAN

ISBN 978-1-957956-20-6 (Paperback)
ISBN 978-1-957956-21-3 (Ebook)

Inquiries and Book Orders should be addressed to:

Leavitt Peak Press
17901 Pioneer Blvd Ste L #298,
Artesia, California 90701
Phone #: 2092191548

Contents

Acknowledgments

WHILE WRITING THIS BOOK IN August 2013, I experienced amazing growth, one that can only be express with words coming from my heart. I'd felt a vacuum in my life because I was grieving over my father's death. One night while meditating and praying before bedtime, I ask my father to talk to me, told him I missed him, and then went to sleep.

During my sleep, I was able to connect with him in a dream. He came to me in my dream and told me to change the format of my book. "Concentrate on what you have learned rather than the pain and bad memories of your experiences," he said. And that is how this book began.

I continued to meditate and connected with myself in ways I did not think were possible. Meditation brought me to a calm state of mind, allowing me to be creative and to learn about myself. In the process of writing this book, I began an experience that let me to better understand my past habits, and the negative images of my thoughts melted away. Writing this book began a self-healing process for me. I can honestly say that it was a miraculous act of God.

My journey has been one of beautiful enlightenment, compassion, and awareness of myself and others. By being open and willing to learn, I can now see what once was hidden. I had to understand that if I wanted to transform my life, I had to rethink and believe in all that I wrote—and practice it. I was willing to follow my inner guide and listen to my spirited being. I began a self-healing process to bring light where there was darkness. I had to let go of the old me and begin anew.

This was a very painful experience for me. Once I released these old images of who I thought I was, I let go and let God take over my life. My transformation began immediately thereafter. I recognized my true potential and understood my need to feel the empty gaps in my life. My self-awareness led me on another journey.

This journey has taught me that no matter the circumstances or the experiences we have lived, it is never too late to change the way we think about ourselves, letting go of the old habits that once held us back. I sincerely hope that you will take my journey to the heart and benefit from your own healing process. It is my deep expression of love that brings me closer to you, the reader. It is the sharing of all my growth and experiences that connects me with you.

My intentions are to help you and guide you connect to your conscious mind so you can find the beauty of your mind power. We all have needs and desires to change, but how we deal with them is what makes a difference in our life. In this book, I sincerely express how I struggle with my way of thinking and how I overcame my subconscious way of thinking to improve my life.

I hope you find encouragement in my words as you go through the path of your own journey.

Frances Mahan

Introduction

Dubai, August 2013. The summer month was not different than the previous one, except that today, during this month of Ramadan, I had decided to participate in a one-month fasting with the local people, the Emirates. It seemed like every other holiday in the Emirates, but August 10 would be a memorable day for me.

Unlike every other ex-pat wife, I decided to stay home instead of travel. It is common for housewives to travel during the Muslim holidays; it is quiet, all restaurants are closed during the day, and most people travel abroad. The ambiance can be overwhelmingly quiet and at times a bit depressing. I had been traveling with my husband abroad for the last eleven years. This year I decided to connect with my inner guide while fasting, and something inside me clicked. Something changed, and I needed to find out what it was. I had found the power of my inner spirit as I felt lost but now, I was found. I once was lost but now was found.

I had struggled all my life with a feeling of wanting something more than just a house, a husband, and all the material things that can make people happy. I had a deep desire to use my gift of expression, writing, through my feelings of separation, death, and sadness. My father had passed away six months before, and I felt as if I was dying inside. Something was missing; I had a big vacuum in my life, and I was eager to determine what was missing.

I needed help but didn't know how to reach out to anyone. I had always been quiet and reserved with my personal issues. I read a lot, loved learning, and found great satisfaction in teaching myself. I joined a coaching study only to find out that I was miserable with the way the person taught. Then I reached out to my own spiritual guide, my divine power, and something great happened. I had found a way to connect at a high spiritual level; I could ask God for anything and see it happen. It was a miraculous discovery.

Chapter 1

WHY DO WE THINK
THE WAY WE DO?

O UR FOUNDATION FOR THINKING STARTS when we are children. We create patterns of thoughts at a very early age from our parents, teachers and loved ones, these thoughts then become our view of ourselves and of others, and they continue to rule our lives until adulthood. We form a perception about who are based upon our thinking patterns. I call it, customary thinking. It's what we are accustomed to think, not what it is.

Our thoughts are stored in our subconscious mind, and we generate these thoughts continuously. The natural Science Foundation (NSA) estimates that we think an average of seventy thousand thoughts per day. The brain has an incredible capacity to store information. It's the most resilient organ there is, but often time, we feel we don't have the power to control our thoughts. "We all do". The brain is made up of 75 percent water, and it stores more information than 1,800 computers. It also uses one-fourth of our blood and oxygen supply. The brain has about one hundred billion neurons, so, if you think you don't have the capacity to change your mind, then think again. You have enough neurons to help you generate energy to think. The brain is one of the most incredible and sophisticated organs of the human body. The brain is the storage of everything we think. Thought empowerment is a great tool of the mind. We all have the power to use our minds to our advantage. We can escape the mental conflict we have created and form a new set of thinking habits. Our healthy thinking habits can increase awareness. First, you must know when, how and why you think the way you do?

Why would you value your thoughts if they are not productive or beneficial to you?

Your thoughts are as important as the credit you give to them. No matter the degree of your thinking, you are responsible for your thoughts. We don't have complete understanding of the mysteries of the mind, and its power to make us think the w0ay we do. Our mind is a complex network of information that relates thoughts between our brain and our conscious and subconscious mind.

I believe there are fundamental limits as to what we know about the mind and its capacities. If you can think about the complexity between the mind, the brain, neurons, cells, conscious and subconscious mind, it is enough to make you wonder. The complete meaning of our life is in our brain. To think that we have one hundred billion cells in our brain is a good indication that our world is not without meaning. The brain and the body are completely different. One cannot see a body without a brain or a brain without a body. The brain works according to the laws of nature, but when we act, we have free will. Our mind chooses what we want. When we make a choice, it is an individual desire. We have the power to change, and to make decisions that impact our lives.

There is a reason why we think the way we do. Our subconscious mind is motivated by fear. Unfortunately, we can sabotage our thinking and suppress our conscious mind. If we want to heal, we cannot allow the subconscious to dominate our thinking, otherwise, our subconscious mind would constantly be in battle with our conscious mind.

We often tell ourselves we don't want to continue thinking these thoughts. Then this thought pattern can appear from nowhere and disappear just as quickly. Your thoughts dominate your life and every opportunity you give them to control your mind. Your thinking can be deeply molded by your old habits because your thoughts are constrained.

Your thinking habits become your reality, and you believe them to be true. They control how you process your thoughts. They even give you feedback about how you should feel about yourself and others. Your thinking habits constantly program your mind, and you then react and think without hesitation. Your subconscious can sabotage the way you think by pulling you back into your old thinking patterns. You must remain aware of your subconscious state of mind. Your subconscious mind can absorb your thoughts at any time. You must build a strong gatekeeper to separate you from the intentions of the subconscious mind or else your subconscious mind will manipulate your thoughts. If you don't take control, you will remain stuck in your mind.

The subconscious mind can be categorized as a computer data programmed delivering information to us as we want it, but sometimes, it gets stocked in the program. Ever wonder why you go from one thought to another, why you're always in constant contradiction with your mind? Well, it is your subconscious mind. Your state of mind is responsible for your confrontations. This mind is responsible for your self-inflicting perception of none reality. It is all about you, your well-being, your sanity and your divine nature. It is you who is responsible for the outcome of thoughts and reaction. Everything outside you can be control by you and how you think.

You have the power and the will to take over control of your thoughts. Your power can take over and defeat your mind's purpose. Anyone who is able to defeat the subconscious mind and enter into reasoning, will understand that the only thing that separates us from successful people, is our perception of our reality.

It all relates to how we have experienced our life, our habits and our thought foundations. Change your thoughts, and you change your mind. Thinking is energy. Our thought process and our neurons work like magnets to hold our thoughts. These magnets dominate our thoughts, our conscious mind, the people around us and all situations. Thinking determines our happiness, and our state of mind, our successes as well as our failures. When we think, we generate a vibration that sends the brain and its neurons signals; these signals produce either positive or negative thoughts, and they are passed on to the subconscious mind for future storage. We then apply them with either fear or courage.

The conscious mind is waiting to grasp at any healthy thoughts, but they are not there, the subconscious mind has taken over. Unfortunately, there is a block between the conscious and the subconscious mind. As a result, the mind blocks all positive thoughts; and the subconscious mind always wins. You then begin to think negative thoughts in every and any given situation. Your thinking habits have now become your reality; you then believe them to be true. But they are not, what you think has nothing to do with your reality; thinking is about how you process your thoughts, what you tell yourself is true about you and the world around you. Reality, on the contrary, is what you observe and make complete sense of. When you are in contradiction with your self or have doubts, there is a constant conflict with your mind; it is a yes or no without a concise answer. These creates an imbalance between your reality, and the perception of what is and is not true. We are the outcome of our thoughts, as the saying…you are what you think. All outcomes in our lives are based on our thoughts. We create the circumstances and everything around us with our thinking. Somehow you find comfort here and don't know how to let go of it. It becomes your place of refuge; a mindset that becomes part of you. You are trapped in an image of a world that seems real to you but is not. It's your own view of it, an illusion of your perception, is an irrational way of thinking. This is not your way of thinking, you have been taught to think this way. You can relearn to think, if you believe in yourself and accept who you are.

Our thoughts are in constant control of our decisions, our actions and judgments. We form patterns of thoughts that dominates our day-to-day actions. When we generate these patterns of thinking, we are constantly facing trials and tribulations. If we continue to worry, then we generate negative thoughts, rewinding them over and over again. We constantly make decisions based upon how we think at that moment. Not a very good habit. We also judge ourselves and others based upon our thought foundation.

If we are critical of others, it is because we have been critical of ourselves. Our thoughts of others have already been formed from the way we think about ourselves. To understand what is going on inside our minds, we must go inward, and reflect outwards. When we use our minds to go inward, the expression of our hearts, minds, bodies and souls is visible to the outside world. We don't need to say much, it is all there! If you connect to these four essentials aspects, your thoughts will reflect your state of mind. You have then transitioned your way of thinking.

If you allow your mind to control your thoughts, then more than likely, your subconscious mind is ruling your thoughts, not you. The good news is, that you can change the way you process your thoughts. You can master the quality of your thoughts, turning them from negative to more healthy and productive thinking. If you can change the present perception of your thoughts, you change the old paradox about the way you have formed your thinking habits. Gradually, you will change your perception about the way you think. The question is, can we really change the way we have being programmed to think? The answer is, yes! You are able to change the way you think, the speed of your thoughts, and your state of mind. You can also re-create the outcome of your thoughts. All this is possible because you have the power to do so. Moreover, this power gives you ownership over your mind. When you take ownership of your mind, you have complete control, because you, as the creator of your own thoughts, have the power to transform the way you process those thoughts. What you feel, think, and know is happening right here, and right now in this moment. Now is all there is, while you are still breathing.

You are not your thoughts, but your life is the product of your thoughts. Everything you think affects you, your family, and your outlook on life. Your thoughts can also affect your health, your productivity, your creativity and your ability to succeed, fail and make rational decisions. Therefore, "Think carefully". and empower your mind with positive thoughts. The power of positive thinking always prevails over negativity. Self-empowerment starts at the conscious level. When you empower your mind, you can fight the negative influences of your subconscious thinking, and you will master your ability to act against unreasonable and poor thinking. You have the power to change the way you think, and so you alone can monitor your thoughts. If you are unable to control your thoughts, then you are the product of your subconscious imagination. Stay positive, appreciate yourself, and improve the quality of your thoughts. Empower your mind and aim for success!

Don't get caught up in mediocrity; don't allow the limitations of your thinking to hold you back from being you. Become the successful, and creative person you are meant to be. Eliminate those unlimited beliefs, and allow your conscious mind to manage your thinking. Think more good thoughts daily. When in doubt, look inwards; this will help you connect to your higher consciousness. Remain positive and empower your mind to focus on your goals.

Recognize your mind's ability to unconsciously rule your thoughts. Know what is going on inside your mind, and understand what triggers your subconscious to think the way it does. Understand when your mind is trying to deviate from your good thinking habits and manage it.

There are times when we feel that we are powerless over the way we think; but science tells us otherwise. Hypnosis can help us tap into the subconscious mind and transform the way we perceive reality and old patterns of thoughts. Transformation is possible when we are able to change and understand the origin of our thoughts. We can recognize why we think the way we do? We control our thinking patterns; and bounce back from our old ways of thinking; shedding the old layer of thoughts for a new, healthy one.

Before you change the old pattern, you must first go through the cycle of thinking habits. Ask yourself, why do

I think this way, what causes it, and get to the core of the problem. Changing your old mind requires that you shift your thinking. This great recording device called, the mind, is capable of multitasking. With awareness, your brain is capable of receiving proper commands from the conscious mind, bypassing the subconscious and tapping into the core of any problem you may have. This is one way of transforming your thinking from negative ideas to healthy and positive thoughts. The truth is that your undivided attention is required to make this happen, or else, nothing will change.

Miraculously, just as your mind can trap you, it can also free you of your mental chaos. When you change your habits, you change yourself—image, your perception, and your ability to deal with everything and everyone that comes your way. Thought empowerment is the answer. The truth is, we don't like to think negatively. We don't want the influence of negative feelings and poor judgments. We don' always think at a conscious level of the mind. That is why our minds are in constant chaos, conflicts and confrontation with our thoughts.

If you feel powerless, helpless and think you don't have control of your thoughts, you will generate more negative thoughts. Until you understand that you, not someone else have the power to change your thoughts, this pattern will continuously repeat itself.

When people feel trapped, they feel as if they have no hope. They monitor their thoughts with the same frequency never changing. As the saying goes, the meaning of insanity is doing the same thing over and over again, expecting different results, nothing ever changes. If you want to live a healthy life, you have to get away from the old, mindset. Live in the now, go with the flow of life, and learn to transform the old, habitual thinking that you have been taught in the past.

Don't live in the past. Today is now, and tomorrow has yet to come. Live in the moment.

We have been taught to think that we are not in control of what we think, that our thoughts are generated by the brain and cannot be controlled. However, we can control what we think. Understanding our thought process, is the guide to changing the way we think. Oftentimes, we are not aware of how our thoughts can affect us. A lack of awareness is like being blind. We constantly move in circles without knowing why. Understanding our thoughts process is the perfect guide to changing the unhealthy pattern we have created in our minds.

Because awareness is the fuel that empowers our mind, keeping it alive and powerful is essential. Thoughts are so powerful that one can compare them to the ability to drive a car. If we accelerate a car and lose control, we will eventually crash. Our thoughts can save us when we need them and they kick in when we are in danger. Survival mode depends on whether we think positive or negative thoughts. If you tell yourself that you cannot make it; you will not, because the subconscious mind has already told your logical mind no! You have now programmed the conscious mind to step away. You have to kick the old habit of thinking negatively and become aware in order to survive. You have to tell yourself, that you can, that it is possible, and you will have the willpower to survive.

The Power of positive thinking can create miracles where there are none. Positive affirmation has miraculous power. You are in control of your thoughts, and your destiny. If you let go, you will be incapable of becoming a happy and fulfilled person. You can become unhappy and developed depression because, you have neglected your true self, the power of your mind. When this happens, you have allowed your subconscious mind to determine your future, and you have lost the power over your minds ability to reason or differentiate, then, depression sets in. Depression is, the neglect of something you want, but cannot get, as well as, the expectations of a false desire. You feel empty, and unsatisfied. Depression is self-denial.

Because our subconscious mind can generate unwanted feelings, you feel let down, and helpless. Hypothetically speaking, the stronger of the two states of mind will always win. Unless you take over, you can find yourself in a very dark place. Depriving yourself of true happiness can lead to depression. People who are depressed find it very difficult to accept help from others. They are alone in a world of their own, making no sense to them. They live in their own state of mind and cannot move on unless, they individually recognize that there is a problem. Acceptance of the truth is the answer. Not even psychological therapy can help them. There are many reasons why people feel depressed, but healing begins with self-determination, with the person wanting to heal. There are instances when prayers are the only answer. I do not recognize any other way you can reach out for help. One must be touched by divine nature, know and trust the reasons for these feelings and beliefs. Surrender completely, and let go and let God.

The good news is that we all have control over our decisions, we are the pilots of our own lives. We learn how to maneuver our own life drama, The possibility of survival or crash, depends on us. Our survival mode in any situation will take over as our thinking kicks in. This is the fight or flight mode. It is all about how and why we think a certain way. Our lives depends on us and us alone.

Only you can save yourself. You cannot ignore your thoughts. Your thoughts-habits will try to interfere, but your awareness will help you ignore and suppress them. Awareness is the key to transformation. With awareness, your consciousness will prevail.

The more you know yourself, the better you are at determining the outcome of your thoughts. You can slow down the thinking with a positive thinking process and change the direction of your thoughts, replacing negative thinking with positive thinking. Its process requires practice; the more you do it, the better you get at it. I refer to this as, an intellectual mental surgical procedure. You have made a complete transition from something you didn't want and replaced it with what you do want.

Our ability to control reality lies within our mental power, awareness, and state of mind. If your thinking is the by-product of what you are experiencing at the moment, then this experience may be gratifying to you. Not only is it good for you, but it's also for your well-being. Your mind is now able to make more wise and rational decisions, and you are free from your old, suppressed thinking. You can also understand that this process is what got you here; and you can now maneuver your thinking habits to remain more balance than before. It is imperative to understand that from time to time, you too will make mistakes and regress to the old ways. Having the necessary tools to fight back is the key to your success. You will know when to cut off the unsolved negative patterns of thoughts, and add new positive things to your mind. You will have cleared old mental blocks from childhood, and you will master your thinking with accuracy and awareness. From now on, the future is yours, if only you dare to dream it! This swift change is the result of your own outcome. You make the transition, thus changing your subconscious believes with your reasoning. Imagine for a moment that you are dreaming, and you know that it is a dream. As you wake up, your awareness of the dream kicks in.

You now know that it was a dream. You are more aware, and you tell yourself, this is not a reality. You control the dream, and you know deep inside your conscious mind, that interpretation of this dream is but an illusion. You have to recognize it as dreaming. Your mind is in a delta state, or you are in a deep sleep, but your dreaming awareness puts you in a theta state. It is as if your mind made the decision to be at two places at one time. Although it seems impossible for the mind to be able to split in two, the fact that it is in a dream state and is aware at the same time, does put the mind into two different states. Do not try to analyze it. Remember that your mind is Quantum, it is capable of being in the past, the present and the future while it is in a dreaming state. The past, because it is dreaming about what happened yesterday, In the future because is dreaming now about an event yet to come and the present because is dreaming now in the present time. The next time you have a dream, and you know that it is only a dream, and remember all the details, this is where you are.

All dreams are but an elusive state of mind, once you wake up, you take over your mind, and you are aware. In order to take over the mind, you go from internal to external reality. Your external reality of how things are, is not free of doubts. The conscious does not always know what it wants. Once you differentiate between these two states, you are in charge of your mental inequality. Your conviction about how you access your thoughts to get what you want, allows you to recover faster. You first must want to make a change. Your intent is sufficient to begin to a healing process.

You may be saying, if only it was that easy? Well, it is! Make the decision, and take initiative, the rest is but the flick of a switch. Healing doesn't happen until you, want to make a change. Your thoughts are your words, and they have all the power in the world. As you think, so you are. You think, then you express who you are. If you are generating negative thoughts; that's who you are at the moment. On the other hand, if your thoughts are directed to positive thinking, then the shifting has begun. Recognize what you are thinking, be aware of that thought, and perceive it as positive in your mind. A thought can only have as much energy as you put into it mentally. It is similar to starting an engine, you first have to put the key in the ignition, and then you turn it on and press the pedal to go. Your command control required an elicit response from the engine and its power.

When you change how you think, your perception and future changes too. You will notice the changes around you and you too will change. In reality, the shift is in you, and because you change, the whole world around you seems to have changed as well. Because you have changed, your world begins to make more sense. You will feel as though, you have opened the door to a world of new opportunities, that had been suppressed inside you. You were not allowing the flow of good vibrations to enter into your life. Now you feel as if a door once locked has just opened.

If a single thought keeps flashing in and out of your mind, you have given negative energy to that thought. The opposite is true about a good flow of thoughts. It is all relative. What you see in your mind, you perceive it and make happen. And you make it happen. When you feel your thoughts have gone out of control, you are angry, stress, or confused, you have handed over your power to the subconscious mind, the ego mind, the mind that resist changes. Once the resistance is over, the nature of your flow is constant and full of good nature. Everything will begin to fall into place.

Know that if at any moment, your thoughts are distorted, then it is time to regain control of your thoughts. If the same thoughts continue, stop and think about where did they have originated, and why? How you handle the situation affects the outcome. It is possible to lose control while you are healing, but that is okay. It is part of the process and requires time, work, dedication, and concentration. If you feel powerless, it is okay, you can always go back to where you started and regain your balance. Know the process, and you know when to stop the mind. Even though it may seem impossible, the mind can use logical thinking when required. The mind is a marvelous facilitator, and it can create miracles. The power is in you to take command of what happens. Positive thinking is the answer! With your mind, you can go from the old to the new as easily as you can think it. That's how quickly it's done. This marvelous inward and outward maneuvering are done with an auto-suggestion to the mind. It changes from the old, bad, and ugly, to the new and beautiful. This is how you master your mind.

Just as the mind can create conflict and chaos with our thoughts, it can also heal you without much struggle. It is a matter of determination.

Although you may be thinking that these mental practices are for people with mental illnesses, you have forgotten the pain and sorrow a person with cancer goes through in their mind. This mental training can help them regain their sanity as they go through recovery. Cancer is not an easy journey to endure physically nor mentally. Having the mental power to endure anything in life is the key to surviving whatever comes our way.

Let us say, one thought originates in your mind of pleasant nature. Your mind will continue or stop! It can instantly recognize that a thought of this nature cannot bring any positive results for your mental outlook. So if you want to improve the state of your mind, you can write down your thoughts. You will change the nature of that thought by instantly recognizing it. Also, you can experience how your thoughts feel, so you bring forth the power necessary to change it after you recognize it. This reasoning will help you recognize the nature of your thoughts. But remember that your thoughts can be deceiving. You will find yourself talking or thinking about something unpleasant that happened to you years ago. Why is that? It is possible to remember what happened to you ten years ago and yet not remember clearly what happened two days ago. If you want to cleanse your mind of old thinking, you can put yourself in a hypnotic state by auto-suggesting changes to the negative vibrations coming into your mind. This is precisely what therapists do, they put you into a positive state of mind to help you change the way you process your thoughts. It is very important that you have faith and conviction in order for auto-suggestion to work for you. Your beliefs, your conviction with less expectations of the outcome will give you more positive emotional intelligence. It will work from the inside out. This will help you erase thoughts that have been dormant in your subconscious mind a long time.

Not only will you balance your mind back to normal and positive thinking, but your belief system will continue to get stronger. The more you face similar situations, the better prepare you will be to handle it. You will notice how smoothly everything will start working for you. If your expectations do not equal your end results, it is simply because you have not put sufficient faith into your thoughts efforts in order to achieve success. Remember that the moment you put your mind into a state of auto-suggestion, the process of transformation has begun. Your mind power is your new tool.

The power of your mind is a main contributor to your mental well-being. We all need to stabilize our thoughts in order to function as normal human beings. It is all about remaining in charge of who we are and what drives us. Mindpower is the balance that prepares you for future success. It is all about how you use your mind to process information, knowledge and common sense. Thought power is the tactic you can use to take over the mind when, your thoughts are out of balance with reality. We must have logic and common sense in order to act prudently and make good decisions. Have you ever met people who are out of balance with their thoughts? They have difficulty making decisions, they always have to ask other people or friends to make the right choices when confronted with decisions. They are uncertain about their own thoughts. If you are unable to control your thoughts, then this means your mind is still not in complete control of your thought faculty. It's time to recognize it and, maneuver your mind in the direction you want it to go. You must take control of your destiny. If you control your thoughts, you will control your destiny. Once the quality of your life has improved, so would your destiny. Thoughts have the power not because we think it, but rather the value we give to them. It is imperative that you know what is going on in your mind. A thought is only a thought because of a situation, people, event, or idea in your life. You give your thoughts energy, vibration and power as soon as they originate in your mind. In order for a thought to process further than the conscious level of the mind, you have to accept and take it to a higher level than when it started. Only you, the receiver, can generate a thought to become a bigger illusion in your mind than it already is. The best solution is to concentrate on one thought and make the best of it. Negative thoughts are an illusion until they become reality because of our impression of them. That is what false thinking is; an illusion of the mind. Thoughts only acquire intensity because we have given them the merits they do not deserve by constantly talking about the same thing over and over. Thus we continue to generate more power, and the thought becomes more real and elusive than before. When you let go of the way you think, you let go of the thought. What you think does not define you. If you are what you think, then think positively. Think good, healthy, and prosperous thoughts. Use the power of your mind to redefine your mental state. When you change your thinking habits, you change your mind, your view of life, and everything around you. You will change the world within you. You can master your thinking habits by renewing your mind with good and healthy information. Read only positive books; inherit good ideas in your mind. You have the right to choose what is good for you. What you read and absorbed makes a significant impact in your mind. Pick ideas and images that will benefit you inwardly. If you can eat healthy food, then you can think and digest healthy information for a healthier mind.

Chapter 2

SHIFT FROM SUBCONSCIOUS TO CONSCIOUS THINKING

O UR MIND WILL RESPOND TO any command as long as you have a strong conviction about what you are doing consciously. The mind can and will respond to your commands. You can practice this with meditation, which helps connect you to the inner source, and helps re-shape the way you use your mind. With meditation there is a calmer state of mind. You will be more reasonable when making decision. During meditation, the mind is in a theta state. What this means is that, the mind is in a state of spiritual awareness, or a dream state. When you meditate or do yoga, the brain cells send signals to the mind. These signals help your mind relax and put you in a peaceful feeling mood. Neurosciences refer to this as coherence or connecting the body, mind, and spirit into one. This feeling gives you a sensation of inner peace, and you begin to think positively about everything. Meditation creates a peaceful sensation and a strong emotional balance to help you overcome difficulties with ease. Because our subconscious mind controls our habitual thought process; it is responsible for how our thoughts are stored and how our mind processes each thought. When we put our mind into a relaxing mode, it is easier to bring it to a more reasonable state, thus eliciting a more positive response as we command with our conscious state of mind. When you find that inner peace, the subconscious mind not longer controls how you think or react. You understand the comfort and can go from a state of disarray, to a calm, relax, and positive state. Your shifting creates positive and creative thoughts. You process thoughts from your conscious mind rather than the uncontrollable subconscious mind. You have gone from operating from the subconscious and to using your conscious mind to command and respond in accordance with your mental state.

How we perceive thoughts

Because we are able to understand the changes in our mind, how we perceive our thoughts changes our mood, and our thinking. These changes in our behavior, help us recognize how we perceive our thoughts. Thoughts are recognize for the value we place upon their meaning. They are neither good nor bad, it is the status we put into them that makes them alive and real. If we accept their nature without judgments, we will be able to appreciate their nature without preconceived notions of the truth.

The subconscious mind perceives thoughts differently than the conscious mind. The reason stands that you feel as though you have lost the ability to trust yourself. Your uncertainty leads you to seek answers outside the conscious mind. You find consensual approval in the mind that supports your insecure comfort zone. The feelings of uncertainty takes over your logic, and fear kicks into your logical state of mind. Your ability to have a clear mind and clear thoughts becomes disrupted by constant doubting and insecurities. You could have a tough time making choices or knowing what you want in life. You are no longer dependant on your own to decide what makes you happy, and you feel stock! Nothing around you changes, and you have no balance in your life.

If you have lost your ability to use rational thinking, you have lost control of your right-minded thinking, then your thought could be deceiving you. In reality, you have lost control of your right-minded thinking. Your thought processes is deceiving you.

Our minds are so complex that we can transform unhealthy thoughts by simply triggering a past experience, which causes the subconscious mind to rule over our thoughts. Thus awareness of the commands, we allow our rational consciousness to be rule. Because everything stars with a thought, the moment we activate a thought, our conscious mind rule over. Our thoughts tells our logical conscious mind to control our thinking unless otherwise interrupted. There is a balance until, our habits infiltrate our mind. Most thoughts are of a healthy nature. It is our perception of them that forms an unhealthy imbalance with the mind. When you are excited about something, your thoughts are in great accord. You are passionate, and in control, and you are a go getter, everything is perfect. All your plans are in order. Then your subconscious mind brings something from the past, and your concentration is deviated to doubtful and questionable thoughts.

Your subconscious mind restrains your conscious mind and attacks your spiritual and emotional well-being. Because it knows how you feel, think, and react, it knows how to block the conscious mind from allowing you to use reasoning.

Your mind can make you feel weak. This feeling of weakness is re-reflected in your thinking, your emotions, and even spiritual well-being. You feel powerless about your feeling, you are not certain of your thoughts, and you project insecurity with an inability to see things clearly. You feel as if there is a lost child inside of you. You are confused about yourself, and your life in general. Your expression, strengths and projections are pure confusion. Nothing seems clear. You act and think based on the demands of others, not your own. You have lost confidence in yourself, consequently, you lose self esteem, and self-worth. You are spiritually un-bound, and will feel as if you don't belong. Your inner child is lost, and you need to connect with it in order to find yourself again.

Often time diseases are simply the end results of our thinking. We create a concept of thoughts that imprison the mind, these thinking habits are created as a set of rules we follow in our mind. A military man who has endured the atrocities of war, knows well these emotions at a subconscious level. They have recurrent thoughts which tortures their mind subconsciously. The quality of our negative experiences out weights our constant thinking and gained momentum as time passes. We constantly feel sick as a result. The mind knows exactly, how you react under certain circumstances, and it will play a game of chess with your conscious. It will keep you sick, confused, and self-destructive, even sabotaging your mind into thinking you are unable and incapable of making decisions. Your subconscious will hunt your thoughts every chance it gets. It owns the way you act, thinking and responding to the outside world as well as internally. These beliefs will make you sick, and illness will appear where there is none. Because the conscious mind is more rational, it takes time to think, and analyze. The subconscious uses your weakness to attack your thinking. If you want to win, you have to believe in yourself, have confidence and be willing. This is done because, you have the power of God and love to practiced with awareness and action.

It is important to understand how the quality of our thoughts can affect the way we process and perceive information. Thoughts originate as a perception of what we believe.

It is inconceivable to think that a simple expression can have a huge impact upon the way one thinks. Wouldn't it be nice if, we could invent a way to erase negative thinking? It would change the way we think completely! But that is not always the case. We are not all so fortunate as to have someone in our lives who is almost perfect to guide us. That someone could impact our lives with impeccable and infallible life rules. It would be magical!

As a teenage, you can find yourself inundated with feelings of sadness, unfulfilled dreams, unhappiness, broken promises and unwanted fears, all because of how you have been programmed to think. You have learned this at a very early age, and now, it is affecting your emotional and mental states. You have to learn to unlock the shackles that are keeping you in the prison of your thoughts. You can do this by changing your thoughts. Learn how to tap into the subconscious mind to find out why you think a certain way. We all have two minds, the conscious and the subconscious mind. One gives instructions, and the other follows. But eventually, one of the two will rule you.

The subconscious mind stored memories and information, and then brings it forth when you ask. Your thinking habits are a decision of the subconscious mind. The subconscious mind tends to resist changes, it doesn't like commands nor directions other than the ones already programmed. The subconscious mind will get you stuck with a habit you do not want anymore, such as drinking smoking or overeating. You the person, have the power to change it by using the conscious mind and bypassing the subconscious. That's not an easy transition because of your thinking pattern, but it can be done. When you have paid attention to subconscious mind conditioning, you can override it to take you where you want to go. The subconscious mind can rule the conscious, but only if you allow to. As you recognize what is going on in your mental dialogue, you will achieve success in making the transition. Remember that the conscious mind is cautious, and patience. This is where you want to be all the time; you need to remain in a steady field of consciousness. This is where awareness resides.

Remember that if you repeat constant learning, your neurons will reconnect. As new neurons reconnect, new neurons will grow new memory, and new cells too. The mind works with a constant repetition of learning generated through the brain. The more you do it, the better you get at it. Remember that healthy cells will pair together and grow to enhance your memory capacity. Life is what we experience, so make your life experience a pleasurable one. Create a set of emotions with thoughts and vibrations, sending them out into the universe with positive energy. Pay attention to your thoughts. Think objectively, and know that your thoughts connect you to God. We are all connected to one mind, but, with our limitation, we create separation.

I am sure there was a moment in your life when, you wanted to change or do something, and you took the initiative. You alone made it happen. We all have done something of which we are proud. Transforming your mind is not different, you simply have to want it. You have it in you, but you have allowed your confused mind to take over your will-power. You have free-will, and are equipped with an inner drive to do the right thing. Unfortunately, you may allow unforeseen circumstances to take control over you. How you will impact your life that made a difference in the world. When you believe in yourself, you feel as though you can bend reality. Your dreams will happen automatically!

When you have taken control over your mind, you will finally know how to improve your thoughts, and you will know and trust yourself. You will feel a sense of comfort inside you. Your intuitions will tell you at what level your mind is operating all the time, and nothing will stand in your way to success. All this is possible because you, the person in need, influenced your thinking with positive conscious re-enforcement. By now, you are thinking from a rational, intuitive self-confident state of mind.

Have you ever made a decision and then changed your mind about it, only to realize you made the wrong choice? This is your intuition talking to you. Your intuition is like your defense mechanism; it always kicks in when you need it. I understand that predicting when your intuition is talking to you is not always easy. Sometimes, our thoughts and circumstances get in the way. Nonetheless, you have free will and can act as you wish anytime.

Learn to listen to your inner self and make better, conscientious choices. If you cannot listen to the voice of your intuition, you will continue to make poor choices. Always stay ahead of what is confusing you inside your mind. Apply what you have learned to help you improve your ability to use the magnificent power of your mind, it will help you defeat the old and move on with the new. Intuition is like your sixth senses, it will warn you when you are in danger and how to get out of it. Or when you are in danger of something. Either. It is like your mental alarm. Learn to listen to your intuitive voice. Intuition is easy when you know what you want, but if you don't know, you will simply hope you understand it.

Repeating the same habits leads to failure. One cannot change nor improve the mind if similar actions, thoughts, and decisions are consistently repeated. You tend to think unrealistically and without reasoning. The mind likes repetition and procrastination. You can get distracted and disoriented with your subconscious thinking; its purpose is to confuse you until it takes complete control of your decisions, choices, and emotions. The subconscious mind take power to change. It adapts easily; you tell it, and it follows. With every effort you make to change your mind, the irrational mind will sabotage you. Irrational thinking takes little efforts. If you are unemployed, seeking for jobs, and consistently get negative feed back from your applications; staying positive is the only rational thing to do. It will try every chance it gets to make you use negative thinking. You will have to change how you think and use more rational thoughts. If you want changes, you first have to listen to your subconscious mind. Understand how and why you are in a constant negative mindset. Why the subconscious mind? Because this is where the problem lies. Analyze your thoughts with reason, and take control of your mind. Break the old habits about how you see things. Understand reality; let go of your confusions about taking action, and build up the strength to do it. Reality is your view or perception about how you see things, people, and the environment. Focus on you, and visualize a new reality.

Thoughts can come into your mind as a result of outside influence, which are then turned into your own perception. Say that a friend or family member calls you and tells you a story about someone who is going through a very depressing time. She lost her father, broke up with her boyfriend, and lost a baby a year ago. If you ever had any of these events happen to you, it is very likely that this will affect you emotionally. Your subconscious mind will immediately go back to a similar event in your lifetime and bring back those memories and emotions. The memories can surface with a similar depressing emotional state as it did in the past. This is a perfect example of how the mind works at the subconscious level. All the negative memories and emotions are stored in it. The mind is like a magnet, it can attract similar energy as long as it is fed with more of it. The more you add to the memory bank, the bigger it gets. Your emotional and mental states of mind have to be balanced. When your brain and your heart are balanced, your thoughts get better, your immune system improves, and your mind is more coherent. Healing the mind is a process. If you are affected by your past thoughts, emotions, and memories, then you are not healed. When you are completely healed, these feelings, thoughts, and memories will no longer affect you. You will talk about it without getting emotional. If you want change or reverse the way you perceive your thoughts, be persuasive with the transformation. Then your decisions and choices will improve. Find the root of your old thoughts. Make good thinking a part of your daily habits. And make it your vision to shine outwards. This is your life journey, and you are in control of the outcome. Make it a wonderful and precious opportunity.

If you resist, life will not help you make things happen. Don't make any drastic conclusion too quickly. When it comes to making decision, the subconscious takes drastic control. You could be thinking about changes and improvements, and then, all of a sudden, a quick doubt impedes your mind. Your mind has just been impacted by an old, familiar habit. It wants to confuse you, and you are unaware of your decisions to act a certain way. This brings nothing but confusion in your mind.

If you resist changes, your mind will control you and you will remain static. Life will only work for you if you allow it to work without resistence. Your past experiences of negative unworthy, judgemental feelings doesn't control your future; you do. Smash the old rules and let life work for you. True happiness doesn't come from what you are, or what you have, it comes from within you. Restore your thinking and find out the real power inside you.

From time to time, I have to stop myself in the middle of a thought. I tell my mind, I have control; I will not let you take over, I can handle it! It may sound crazy, but it works. You have to stop the process before it gains any strength and disrupts your mind. Remember that your thoughts are not who you are. They are not your life story; they are the by-product of what, how, and why you think the way you do. But all that can be change. You can change how you perceive your thoughts. Your thoughts are your beliefs about yourself and others, and they are not always a reality. You are responsible for your thoughts. When you think about something or someone, you are making preconceive assumption about it. The reality unfolds only when you find out the truth. Your thoughts are not always reasonable, correct or real. Whatever you think, and perceive about it, you are the product of it. I am sure you have heard the expression. "The first impression is what counts". Well, not always. Depending upon the state of mind of an individual, first impression can either be gracious or unpleasant. Lets say two people just got separated or divorce. Would they be very cheerful, happy and outgoing? Not likely. But when you meet them, your image of them has been formed. You have made an assumption based upon your own judgment of what you saw. This is only your perception of the truth, not the reality of it. Reality is action, while an illusion is a dream, an imagination. Illusion is a rejection of the truth. "The first impression is what counts". Well, not always. Depending upon the state of mind of an individual, first impression can either be gracious or unpleasant. Lets say two people just got separated or divorce. Would they be very cheerful, happy and outgoing? Not likely. But when you meet them, your image of them has been formed. You have made an assumption based upon your own judgment of what you saw. This is only your perception of the truth, not the reality of it. Reality is action, while an illusion is a dream, an imagination. Illusion is a rejection of the truth.

Likewise, when you feel rejected, unloved, it is because you have created that belief system into your subconscious mind. You believe that to be true but, once you change your view on how people feel about you, your thoughts will be different. It is not how you perceive others feel about you, but rather, how you feel internally about yourself. As you think, so you are. You created the mood, and the intention of your internal dialogue in your mind. You alone belief this thoughts to be real, no one can make you feel this way. But you believe that your feelings are being hurt, that your heart is broken, and that others have no respect or love for you. You need not find the answer inside you. If you look deep within yourself, you will find that the answer has always been there. You have chosen to neglect yourself, and your love, feelings, emotions, acceptance, respect, and individuality. You have always been loved, but you don't see it. Others cannot give you what you don't already have. It all starts with you!

All is well if you find what you are looking for deep inside you, not in others. When peace, love respect, purpose, and the need to help reside in you, then all your questions have been answered. Change begins with you. If you listen to your gut feelings, your intuition, and your instincts, you will be your own best friend. Shift your paradigm and find out how to think differently. The good news is that if you shift the perception of your thoughts, you will accept your thoughts to be different than what you have previously believed. You will be happy, and happiness will create your success. To find true happiness, do what you love. You will need positive stamina to bounce back from where you are and remain happy not matter the outcome.

It is not the experience of a particular thought that matters but rather, the conscious or subconscious reality you attribute to it. If you grew up with the inflicted thought that you are not good enough for anything, your perception about how you feel about yourself can affect you tremendously. But if you ignore the thought, and fight for what you as an individual believe about yourself, the sky is the limit. Only you can limit your thoughts and your ability to function in life. There is not such a thing as I can't! Remember that you can use adversity to your advantage. You can triumph or your can constantly follow in misery. The question is, which one would you prefer?

When you begin to adhere a new way of looking at your life, then your future and your mental state, will follow. All it takes is a firm decision to follow your gut feelings and thoughts. You need to know what makes you feel good, and what causes you to feel unhappy? It is all in the balance of knowing the difference. Then you can focus on making a new direction in your life. It takes time to transition internally, when your state of mind is heading in the right direction with your guidance. You begin to create positive energy, and change your thoughts, which helps you release all the quilt, negativity, and resentments. Implant new beliefs in your mind. When you do, you operate from a sense of certainty, and a state of consciousness. You will reflect outwards into the world with a higher lever of emotional confidence. Your dreams will happen automatically. As a result, your progress, and your view of future will be the products of your internal, and external state of my mind. Set your goals to be different, but challenged yourself to do what you thought was impossible. You will accomplish, if you commit. With a clear mind, you can take any habits, judgments and thoughts, and silence the negative mind and thus become a winner. You will become detached from the negativity of your past, and you will embrace the future with a positive attitude. Your energy helps you detach from the old and, release new patterns of thoughts. This is a good way to cleanse your thinking. The aim is not to concentrate only on what you are trying to achieve, but to connect to your conscious mind and reject old habits. You connect to your true identity, reject unwanted thoughts, and cleanse the way you have been reacting. If you think it cannot be done, think again! If your brain can process 25,000 billions of thoughts per second, then imagine what power your mind has. Focus on your intent to improve your mental state. Don't judge yourself for the outcome of your trials; let go of the assumptions that life is what you want it to be. Work with your inner strength and bring a magical straightforward transformation.

The mind has an extraordinary power to receive, and exchange information. Don't resist change, all you need is to have conscious awareness of your thoughts. Change your confusion about reality to view things as they are. Use your vision, imagination, and inner silence to help you concentrate on your goals. Use the power of your mind to concentrate on your intentions. Use gratitude as a way of valuing your life. Read positive books, relate with people who share your dreams and values, remain focused, and be grounded. Humbleness and humility will get you a long way, don't be afraid to be natural, to be yourself, as you are.

The nature of the mind is to think healthy thoughts. We all want to be nourished, to be appreciated, to be balanced. But sometimes circumstances, people, and events interfere with our lives. Quite often, we go on a different tangent, our minds get distracted, and reality is not what we perceive it to be. We then end up in a big mess, and our lives are in complete confusion. You can go from thriving to feeling like there is nothing significant in your life. You can feel stuck.

Then, one day, something hits you, and you shift your conscious mind from not having hope to wanting to make a difference in life, it is human nature to be kind, to give and to want to help, but it is easy to get distracted and lack empathy. The mind can turn 360-degrees and change from one state to the next, just like that! This is how the mind works. We still don't know the full extend to how the brain works. Much research is needed in neuroscience to fully understand the nature of the brain, the mind, and our capacity to process thoughts.

Your moods and emotions can be sending signals to the mind that you need to make a change, and so you will experience resistance from the subconscious mind. Again, this means your old habits need to be desensitized from the subconscious mind, and you should focus all your attention on the conscious mind. The temporal lobe in your brain is constantly retrieving old imprinted memories from the past. The good news is that we don't have any limits to how far the human brain can be trained. We only know that as science continues to search, we learn more about the brain. The more we experience, the more we learn. New findings are been discover everyday. It is important to understand the balance necessary to change how we feel, as we experience our thoughts. When we understand the balance or unbalance of our minds, we absorb energy from thoughts, and energy from our collective memory. We constantly reflect on the past to talk in the present, thus, revising emotions that would eventually impact our minds. Most of the time, these thoughts are not of healthy nature, and quite often, we go back into our childhood memories to reflect on good times. We have a tendency to want to talk about what we have done, because, that is how we identify who we are. I did this, and I did that. Even as we grow older, we reflect on the things we no longer have. We trained our mind as a plug that connects directly to areas of our life past events whenever we bring a thought forward. The subconscious mind is programmed to relate in the past then, we feel the need to reform with what is more familiar to us at an unconscious level, rather than conscious.

When the mind is more active at a subconscious state, we are practically operating without a conscious awareness of our reality. When we operate from this level of the mind, we deprive ourselves the joys of life, and there is no peace within. Nothing is real, all is threatened, and there is not peace within us.

If you can understand the nature of your thoughts now, chances are, you will know exactly how to manage your thought patterns. You will be aware of what thoughts to allow and which ones to let go. As you manage your thinking, things will be different. By now, you have established a method of self-improvement with your mind that will last you as long as you remain coherent with your thoughts. But your awareness at a conscious level is required; know that your subconscious mind will try to resist your progress. You must stay focus.

Remember that the more you practice, the faster your brain will master at tasking the problem.

Knowing that you are the master of your thoughts is a powerful feeling. We all have it, but not all of us can master it easily. Build your future based on your present, and the healthy ideas of what you want from life. Renew your mind, and rewire your brain for success. Be free from all the fragmented concept of your subconscious ideology.

Focus on defeating your old beliefs. Become more self-conscious of your subconscious ability to interpret your thoughts, and don't let it sabotage your creative ideas. Furthermore, it is good to know, that you don't have to act or think in accordance to the demands of your subconscious mind. You have the choice to be or not to be. Protect yourself, don't allow negative thoughts to rule your life, your future, and your projection of life. This lifetime belongs to you, don't go back into the past to reflect on it.

Awaken your mind, and use your intellectual energy to be more creative with new ideas to make a positive impact in your life, and to flow freely. As you let go off the limiting beliefs, you create a new state of mind. Don't allow your past or bad habits to rule your future endeavors. Rather than giving up and feeling helpless, contribute to more positive energy in your thoughts. You will be able to influence, empower, and recondition your mind. You can learn to process basic common sense, take on new tasks, and master every thought that comes to your mind without having to use your irrational mind. The past is gone, and today is now! The future is yet to come, so act for today. Empower yourself and the world around you. The majority of our thoughts are illusive, we spend half of our time thinking rather than doing. Over-thinking destroys our mental energy, rather than make us feel accomplished. We all want to be fulfilled in life and no take our dreams to the grave. To be successful at mastering the mind, we have to recognized the impact our thoughts have on us and in our daily lives. Creative constructive conscious thinking is the goal, but with a subconscious re-evaluation.

Of course we don't go to the subconscious to fix the conscious mind, rather, we eliminate old habits we have created in our subconscious mind, and we change the way we think. We tap into the subconscious to renew our present perception of our thoughts. Without the mental clutter, our thinking will become clear. We go into the subconscious mind and stop the process of thought before acting or saying anything. We first have to face the gatekeeper; the subconscious mind. By changing the blueprint of the subconscious mind, we are able to perform better. We now operate from our conscious state of mind with a steady, healthy, and more productive state of mental outlook. We become one with ourselves and all we do. We master our destiny, projections, and perception, but most of all, we create all that comes to us. Magical! That is the power of the human mind.

Moreover, when we understand that change does not happen overnight, we will make the necessary efforts to allow change to happen. Dreams cannot be achieved if, we set standards too high, if we do, we will fail, and the old pattern of behavior will set in again. The truth is that we spend half of our life-times thinking.

The majority of our thoughts are more illusive than not. As a result, we create unhealthy habits, and healing takes longer. To maintain a healthy state of mind, we must start thinking positively. But first, we should give ourselves credit for starting. It all starts with an effort to want to transform our mind, rather than stay in the unhealthy unworthiness of our thoughts.

Understand that you are trying and do your best. Even spiritual professionals in the field of self-help are working on improving themselves. It is a learning process. Our thoughts can be restored as long as the individual is willing to work. The process to heal the mind is different for each person. For some, it takes the simple use of meditation and hypnosis, for others, the healing process is more lengthy, difficult, and painful. The difference is based on the trauma experienced by each individual adult or child, or how we spend half our lives worrying and thinking unhealthy negative thoughts. The majority of our thoughts are wasted into creating dreams we never conquer. We make plans to start a project or take a course, and then, we find plenty of excuses to not finish. We are creatures of habits. Sometimes, we set our- selves up for failure. We buy clothes we never wear, and waste money unnecessarily. We do the same with our state of mind, we put it on standby, wasting precious time and energy. We procrastinate, and don't allow changes in our lives. No wonder we feel emotionally stock sometimes.

Not only do we have to think positively and take action, but, we have to stop the cycle of unhealthy thoughts. If our thoughts are not productive, then they are unhealthy.

To change the way you think, you have to train your mind to think with more compassion, kindness and love to self and others. The moment you take charge, you will be free, relieved and non-judgmental. You will let go of your ego and act with a more empathic heart. Know that today you have the power to change the way you think, and think new healthy thoughts. Your thoughts will empower you to make a difference in your life. When your conscious mind has taken over, the weak mind has not choice but to follow. Consciously, you have achieved success, and have reshaped your mind to think the way you want.

To help you understand how the quality of your thoughts affect your mind, I first must walk you through the process of healing. Now, lets get deeply into the mind, and understand why we think the way we do. When you dream, you go deep into a delta state of mind, in this state, you are relaxed. Nonetheless, your mind and your brain are still in processing information. It is during this state that the brain is most active. Think for a moment about the fact that even in this state, you are able to record and remember what and how you process information from your dreams. What this means is that the brain sends signals to the mind, and our memories are stored. Then, just as easy, the brain brings them out when necessary.

Chapter 3

GIVE YOUR MIND THE
COMMANDS YOU WANT

D ON'T ALLOW YOUR MIND TO drive you crazy; take command of your thoughts. Your mind has an incredible capacity to take commands, and it can change from its present state to any state you command. Let me explain that further. When a person sleepwalks, he can be asleep and get up in the middle of the night, do some housework with his eyes open, and not remember what took place the next day. This gives you an inside look into how powerful the mind is. The brain controls your subconscious mind during sleep, and sends signals to the mind as if you are in a state of hypnosis. You can be asleep but functions as if you were awake. What this implies is that your mind has taken command from the subconscious to act, even though you are asleep.

The brain is responsible for generating fresh ideas and creativity, and sends signals to the mind while we are asleep. This simply means that the brain is more active while we are asleep. Our thinking process accelerates. Think back to the analogy of the car accelerating out of control. The mind never stops. Our thoughts are constantly generating, even when we are resting. We dream, and we remember details, images, and everything that happened. But how is that possible? Although, our dreams happened at a conscious state of the mind, the subconscious mind plays an important part in recording the dream for us to remember. You can think of your subconscious as a predator of your thoughts, an imposter or an alternate illusive state of the mind, sometimes, not always. Your subconscious mind can distract your thoughts even when you are not completely awake. The reason why we remember our dreams is because they have been stored in the storage of our subconscious mind. This is why we react when those memories are recalled. They are like images recorded in our memories or subconscious mind. When we access them, we react to an external negative illusive demand. Our memories can be pleasant or unpleasant, the results depend upon our present state of mind. But there is hope: we don't have to react nor respond to the old demands of the subconscious mind.

When you are dreaming, you can wake up and tell yourself that is only a dream, and then you can continue dreaming as if nothing happened. Think healthy thoughts before bedtime; this will increase the possibility of having pleasant dreams. We can take control of our thoughts, believe that we are not the by-product of our past and begin to think more clearly. The ask ourselves, what thought brought this to mind? Do I need to process this or let it go? You decide how to command your mind. How does it want to enter my mind and why? Once you can ask yourself these questions, you will begin to understand the reason and origin of your thoughts. It has been said that thoughts can move mountains, motivate you, and create the reality one wants. You are in control of everything you think. You, the creator of your thoughts, can make your world the way you want it. This is how you create an image of what you want to become. One single thought has enough power to change your life from misery to prosperity, from sadness and despair to happiness, and from depression to light, life, love, and spiritual well-being. Your view and perception of what you and your life truly mean do not depend on the views of others but rather on your own. When we think, not only do we generate energy, but the vibration sends waves of transmission into the universe that multiply those vibrations back to us. Be careful what you think, your thoughts have power. They can manifest anything into a reality. Your thought energy can work with you or against you, so, think positively to increase the level of energy of your thoughts. Take command of your thoughts. When your thoughts are of lower vibration, there is no energy to help you carry them through. Imagine that you want to win the The California Lotto, you put much effort in thinking about it, play every week, and ask God to help you win. Then, you think, when will I win, why not me, and so on...you don't let go of the thought of winning day and night.

You use all your positive energy and good frequency thinking about one thing. Realize that if you let go and allow it to manifest into your life, all things are possible. It is the amount of attention you have used to make it happen that had not made it happen. Relax and let go, believe that all is well, and you will win.

When you control what you think, you give power to the conscious mind, not your subconscious mind to act on your behalf. Allow positive thoughts to flow with good vibration, then your mind will release any unwanted thoughts creating a new vibration for thinking. Then you watch your mind in action. Study your mind's shift and make modifications where needed. Make observations as to how you behave when familiar conditions are presented to you, then you will manage to let go of your old mental state.

If you carry memories from childhood that were taught to you by a family member, using a form of punishment in you, chances are, the next time you are presented with a similar situation, you will begin to feel the sensation of the old memories. You now associate your past negative experience with this present state of mind. Talk yourself into understanding that you are now a different person, and that past cannot affect how you feel. Mentally put a stop to the old perception of what you used to believe. If you approach things with diligence, the problem will disappear. We all have the willpower to make good choices that can benefit us. Say to yourself, "I am the answer. I can, and I will transform how I think today."

Let's say, a friend says something you find offensive. You either contribute to her thinking, or you let go and forget that she even said it. Is not up to you to change your friend, but you can separate yourself from things that are not healthy for you. You can differentiate because now you are able to think more rational. You do this with compassion and understanding for the other person. When you use reasoning, it gives you a sense of well-being, self-gratification and understanding towards others. Thinking is internal power and energy reflected outwards.

The fact that you can choose how you think can help you reform how you use your mind to your benefit. You believe that you have the strength to understand what is going on in your mind. Know what makes you think the way you do. Why the doubts? Why the constant submission to the subconscious demand? Why does it take so long to recognize that you have the power in your mind to improve the way you think? Sometimes you get stuck in your old ways, and you believe that your life is not under your control. You hand over your power to the game of life. You follow along with the flow and forget you have a bigger problem; figuring out what is wrong with your way of thinking.

Each sequence of events that unfolds during your lifetime is like an elevator. How you interpret and manage each floor on your way up, will determine the outcome. In your pursuit of happiness, you either reach high or low. It is part of the flow of life. The outcome of the journey is entirely up to you. Tell your mind what kind of thoughts you want to have; don't wait for God or your subconscious to think for you. Rather, give your mind a command. In order to take over your mind, you have to bypass all the false expectations you have about your subconscious and make the right decision. Use your power of persuasion and take a leap of faith with your thoughts. You need to understand that your thoughts are actions, and the reaction of it is part of your perception. You either accept or reject them depending on how you reason, you weigh out the benefit they will have in your life. If you get stuck in your thought process, you will reap what sow. Taking over would make a significant difference in your life. When the mind game changes, you will need a new set of rules to follow; then you can play the game of life with honesty and integrity.

When we are in a difficult or critical life situation, our thoughts and actions can be the only key to our survival. Thinking is critical because it plays a very important role in how we make decisions when it comes to life and death. We can pull ourselves out of any situation by using the power of our thoughts. Our chances for survival can also be sabotaged by our state of mind; how we react during critical circumstances depends on how we perceive our chances for survival in our mind, or how our capacity to pull out of any situation helps us shift our thoughts. It is called, "thoughts power".

Let's say you get stranded in the middle of the sea with no drinking water, and no food; you only have a raft to keep you afloat. You are at sea for four weeks. You are weak, pale, dehydrated and hallucinating about your life. Thoughts about your life come and go. Would you give up? or would you have hope that somehow, you will be rescued? How you think will depend on your chances for survival. Your incapacity to think positively will shorten your chances of you staying alive. With positive thinking you can overcome the impossible and make things happen. Your ability to think positively will enhanced the vibration of your thoughts to make things happen for you. As you encourage yourself to think positive all the time; your thoughts will work with you, not against you. If you are convinced that an idea or thought is what you want, then remain positive no matter the outcome, and things will happens because your subconscious mind is not working against you anymore.

People sabotage their thoughts because they don't have a firm belief in what they think or want. Accepting failure rather than success is not your preferred choice; don't postponed your goals and dreams because of your beliefs. Instead, take over your life and your decisions to receive all that you deserve. Use the power of your mind.

Have you ever wanted to buy a house so badly that you did all the financing required, and you dreamed about living in the house, and talked about it all the time, but for some reason it does not manifest for you? You don't get approved. You ask yourself, "I have done everything, and still, nothing! Why?" You have unconsciously doubted yourself! One single thoughts has created a ripple of negative energy which created a negative outcome. This is the end result of negative thinking.

When it comes to decision-making, self-doubt is the only thing standing between you and what you desire. Let your thoughts flow with ease as they are meant to. If you interfere, you will have a difficult time understanding the outcome. Attract what you want in your life with your mind. Use this power to your benefit.

Situations and events are already predetermined by the way we perceive them in our mind. People refer to this as the law of attraction. This is the power of your mind at its best. How you imagine and manifest what you want in your mind will be super-energized by the power of your thoughts.

Our mind never stays silence. We need to learn how to silence the mind to help us make things happen without distraction. Oftentimes, we send vibrations into the universe about something we want, but we don't know how to keep our inner voice silence. *We think, what if? Can I? What would happen if?*

Unfortunately, this is the way people think. That's why you have to train your mind to allow the moment to unfold without you trying to make it happen. To truly experience the power of your mind, you need to know what drives you to do something with passion. How does it feel for you to achieve success? How do you attract what you want with your mind? Is there a sense of control that helps you envision and project what you want? Or are you driven by some internal force in you that gives you a feeling of certainty and security? Perhaps it's all of the above. When you have power within, there is a feeling of certainty that cannot be stopped. Nothing can stand in your way. Your intuition, your mind, your body, and your spirit work together. Learn to listen to your inner voice have faith in what you know, pay attention to your feelings, and allow your body to feel the empowerment. It is a marvelous experience.

The better you know yourself, the better you will handle any given situation. The power of your mind becomes a form of self-preservation for you. Being self-conscious is the key to creating empowerment within. This helps you become mentally strong with a confident in mastering your mind, and create anything you want in your life. You then become the true authentic self-conscious hidden person in you. You have now master the task at taking full command of your mind.

Reshape How You Think

If you ever had a project to complete or a new job, and your mind seems to be preocupied with thoughts and worries, this is a good indication that you are having difficulties making a choice or reasoning about your thoughts without worry. Or you are uncertain about which direction to go. The best choice for you is to reshape the way you are thinking and create a new pattern of thoughts. This will help you clear your mind and start fresh. Taking a nice walk, meditation and fresh air helps release the clutter in your mind. Something will eventually give. New thougths will emerge to help you decide what is the best way for you to move in a different direction. You control the outcome of your own programming mentally. You alone reshape how to think constructibly for your benefits.

Once you reshape how you think, you can make the intelligent choice to stop the impure thought process, and take over your mind control? You have to liberate your thoughts of old paradigm in your mind. You need to fly above the storm of your old thinking and create miracles where there are none. You must heal at all three levels, spiritually, mentally, and consciously to create a change in your mind for the better.

How we process our thoughts has everything to do with how we reshape our mind. How we perceive the world to be creates an image about it in our mind. What you think has already been accepted into the mind before you can analyze it. Is the capacity of the mind to absorb information that allows thoughts to become a reality? Sometimes fear plays a big role in how you shape your thoughts, you either allow things to become present in your life, or you stop the process from evolving by presenting fear as an obstacle. Fear can lead you to become guilty, judgmental, and self-critical unless you re-shape the way you think.

The more you repeat this behavior, the more difficult it becomes for you to restore your thinking. You will struggle with your mindset. Reshaping the mind takes a logical acceptance of false beliefs. A good example is, if you ask your best friend or husband how do I look? And one says nice, but the other says not! Which one would you believe? Or are you going to use a self-conscious approach at the truth of what is to make a decision based on it? You already know the answer. But you go outside of you to find it. The solution is not based on the multiple choices you have, rather the awareness you have about your individual decision that would affect you mentally and emotionally. Understanding why you doubt your self is important for progress.

Giving your mind the commands you want to reshape how you think means that you have a complete understanding of what is going on in your subconscious. You now control your mind, your thoughts and their flow. You tell your mind whether to generate positive or negative thoughts. You know how to do this because you have the power to recognize whether any particular thought is beneficial to you and your well-being. What has taken shape here is not necessarily your mind, but it is actually your conscious logical thinking. You control, make choices, accept the responsibility, take courage, and initiate it with a new state of mind. Restructuring how you think is about the mind, how you process information, how you perceive thoughts, and how you recognize the nature of your thoughts.

You can reshape your mind, if you know how to manage your thinking. You can control what you think, and let go of the negativity and confusion of your subconscious mind with repeated mental practices. Becoming aware of what you are thinking creates self-discipline in your mental processing daily. Practice before you speak or say something. Stop, regulate your thoughts, pause for a moment, then say what you are going to say slowly. This practice will help you rewire your thinking before you speak. You are depending on yourself to rewire the way you think. You alone have taken charge of the circumstances by which your subconscious has control over your mind. When you draw mental positive energy into your life, the results of your vibration will multiply with more energy. Yes, you can redefine the dogmatic state of your mind, and yes, you can do it alone. Often times professional help may leave you more confused because your state of mind is so devastated that you cannot see right from wrong. You allow your thoughts to take over your mind, and you don't recognized what is happening. You talk about the same problems and situations all of the time. Then, you read a book or watch a show on T.V. that points precisely to your problem. An eye opener. You recognize the problem. You take over and reshape the way you are thinking. It takes a small effort and lots of trials, but it can be done. You let go and let God guide you through it. You are powerless until you take control.

To overcome any adversity in life, you must be balance with a spiritual, mental and peaceful heart flow. Know that internal and external influences are also important because they keep you mentally balanced. To make this transition of reshaping your mind, you must first know who you are? It is there, you just have to find it. Then your life will be molded into something of true meaning and purpose with magical power. Everything in life is relative; you have to understand the process by which the law of the universe spells things out to you. It is there, you just have to find it. Then your life will be molded into something of true meaning and purpose with magical power.

There are times in our life when we seek for answers that are only a thought away from our understanding. Yet circumstances, and events that happened in our life's can lead to mental trauma, which can derail the logic of our thinking. The lost of a loved one, an accident, mental or physical abuse, war, or a mass shooting can be the causes of such traumatic experiences in our life. Nonetheless, there are no right answers or solutions to healing our mind from pain or trauma. We all have to learn and experience through our own mental journey of what it means to be a self-conscious rational thinking human being.

You connect to your higher self, radiate from within, and life takes a different meaning. Your mind set is aimed at helping rather than asking for help.

There is a saying about purpose; purpose is giving birth to your natural gift because it wants to express itself through you, the receiver.

Chapter 9

What Is The Purpose of Our Thoughts?

AKE A MOMENT TO THINK about what an ideal day looks like for you. Next, know that if, you can dream it, you can achieve it. Your mind has the power to create what you want. Therefore, the purpose of your thoughts is to use them constructively, and to your advantages. The purpose of imbalanced thoughts is to confuse you, create chaos and deplete the energy you have in your conscious mind. Think and beware! Your thoughts are in constant inequality with your mind, whether it is your subconscious or your conscious mind. Your mental balance is the main issue. Unless you, take control of the imbalance you have created, your purpose in life can be defeated. Then much effort needs to be put into transforming your thinking. Instead, create a sense of well-being and stay focus.

When you pursue your purpose in life, your happiness and destiny will unfold for you. If you lose your momentum or mental balance, you will feel as if your purpose is wasted. You will not feel any sense of gratification, rather you feel let down by your own failures. Pursue your purpose, happiness, destiny, and how you balance your well-being. If you lose your mental balance, you will feel as if your purpose is wasted. You will not obtain your goals, and you will feel let down by your own. The idea of thoughts is not to create illusions, but to understand how to process what we are thinking and use it to our benefits. Healthy thinking aligns us with our purpose, and help us influence others in a positive way. You have learned in the previous chapter how to command your thinking and control the quality of your thoughts. Think about how important it is to maintain your mental equilibrium, If you were a teacher, a Doctor, an Astronaut, or a Pilot. It is imperative to have his quality in any of these professions. Therefore, it is no different in you. Our thoughts have a purpose and it is to use them to the best of our mental capacity not matter who you are.

As you recondition your thoughts, you will begin to make a big impact on the way things manifest into your life. With the control of your mind, you will project and allow things to occur with more confidence, purpose, and a healthy positive sense of reality. Because you have allowed your consciousness to take a magical direction, you have opened a new door of possibilities. It's that simple! Your ability to see the world around you from a different perspective has helped you create a new image of your- self. You have created a strong bond of energy between your mind and your conscious thinking. This is referred to in psychology as collective conditioning thinking. As a result, you are more aware of what you are thinking, all the time. You have changed your thought patterns and thus inherited a new way of processing information with your thoughts. This is the purpose of thought balance, you objectively chose what is of value for you.

People tend to forget that their goal is to improve the quality of their thoughts and share the benefits with others. Sharing is contagious. The more you know, the more you want to share with others. I refer to this ability of the mind as ultra intelligence; It is the ability to tap into the highest level of your intellect, condition your thoughts, process information from your brain, and then share the experiences. People who meditate claim this is how they connect to their intellectual intelligence, their guide and their God. They listen to their inner voice.

When we meditate, it allows the physical body to remain calm, the mind connects to the unconscious higher intellect, goes deep into consciousness, and remains there. This is then reinstated into the external with a more powerful sense of perception, intelligence, peace and calmness. This may be a bit confusing if you don't meditate. This state of consciousness is possible for anyone who wants to connect to a higher level of the mind. Not matter the circumstances, it can be done. What you are doing is conditioning the mind to follow the peaceful direction you have selected, thus maintaining a good balance with your thoughts. Furthermore, you learn to listen to your inner silent voice, the voice of spiritual awareness between you, your soul and your guide or God. Think of it as having sensory perception, it takes a very deep mindset to reach this level of the mind. One can experience, feel, and imagine with the mind. The actual connection between all three is your ability to see and feel things that are not there but do exist. The mind is capable of experiencing an existence that is neither physical nor real. It is as if you connect directly with God. And if God exists in our imagination, then everything else is possible. It is all about how the mind interprets the experience and the connection. It is all about that inner voice that speaks to us in silence.

Now that you have balance in your thinking, listen to your inner voice, and believe it is possible to connect to your higher level of mind intellect. Doing it is a matter of practice, this is also part of self-awareness. I know this formula very well. Self-awareness is a constant reminder to keep yourself focus on your daily thinking. It is an integral part of everyday living. I have done it, experienced it, and practiced it many times. You can listen to many videos, and purchase many products to help you, but, unless you believe that you can make it, you will continue to be exactly where you are. We have to learn to listen to our inner voice to regain our mental confidence, and be self-conscious about what is coming out of the mind as a thought. Before you go to sleep, chances are you are having a recollection of thoughts as a reflection of your day. Take notice of the thoughts you are having. Create a pattern to change your thinking, pray, take a deep breathe or count from 1 to 10. This will break the pattern of thinking before bedtime. Know that you can defeat mental all obstacles, because you have the power to control what is going on in your mind.

We have reached a new age, and are becoming more and more self-conscious.

We have learned that we are at one with all that is in this universe. Or we are one with the universe? Which one? If you put your energy and desires out into the universe to manifest, then it will. Energy equals frequency and manifestation. Because we are vibrational energy, and we are incorporated into the energy of the universe, we can manifest anything with our mind-brain energy. You simply have to allow things to evolve for you. Your purpose is projecting what you want. Ask, and you shall receive. Allowing it and releasing it into the universe will allow your desires to manifest for you. It is like the law of karma: you get what you put into it. Therefore you have to learn to value your thoughts. You must know and differentiate positive from negative thinking. Value your thoughts as you value yourself, and know that you get exactly what you ask for. If you need more, then ask for more; don't limit yourself. You are your own limitation!

Now that you know your purpose and the value of your thoughts, you will maintain a balance between your mind and your consciousness. You have all the resources needed to make reasonable and healthy choices that will enhance the fruit of your spirit. Using consciousness within consciousness and divine timing will produce success in you. Once you do, your purpose had begun, you can now enjoy the fruit of your hard mental labor. Every day you awake, you will engage a mental state of positive thinking. You will project and send signals to the universe to work for you, as well as your desired goals with good intentions. Believe that as you value your thoughts, you don't have to confine yourself to the demands and needs of others. You now value your thinking in order to make wise choices. The inner voice you didn't know before now communicates with you at a very deep level of your conscious mind. You are now the director of your life drama. There is a voice deep inside your mind. One can see it in the movies when a subconscious mind speaks to the conscious and guide one's thinking. This inner voice is like another persona, it can also be referred to as the crazy mind, because if you talk or think like this, then you are crazy! But isn't that the case with mind control or even a constant repetition of our thoughts? Our thoughts are not always rational because our thoughts determine our rational or irrational way of thinking.

For instance, have you ever had an idea that was so crazy you didn't want to share it with anyone? Then one day, you watch a movie or a television program, and your idea is being projected? We all have crazy ideas and crazy voices in our mind, but that is how new inventions and possibilities are created. Of course some thoughts are crazy in nature, but if you want to know how to interpret your thoughts, then learn to analyze what is coming in your mind and make good sense of it. Your ideas can become part of your future dreams, and they can change your reality overnight. Don't ever underestimate the power of your inner voice speaking to you. Control the voice of your thoughts, and manage your life in the right direction. It is not what you think but rather how you process it.

These voices are not always rational. Your intuition will let you know. I am sure you have experienced heart palpitations or a feeling of something you cannot understand. You think something is wrong with you, or you feel as if you are losing your mind. These feelings persist on. These are the voices in the minds of an alcoholic or drug user. They experience voices in their head from the hallucination of drugs or alcohol overdose. They either have an aha moment or figure out exactly what is going on. Sometimes, they speak as if it is not them, but the voice of an altered state of knowledge in their subconscious mind. This voice is their inner being talking from their guts, and intuition or the voices of their inner demons. Our conscious higher intelligence knows more than we think.

This state of the mind that we don't completely understand is our pure conscious intelligence, the rational mind.

For example, when we make a decision and the results are not as favorable as we expected them to be, we learn from them. But when we don't pay attention to our feelings and our intuition, we end up overanalyzing things or bypassing the true meaning.

The same cannot be said for the inner voice which speaks to us from the subconscious mind. This voice does not speak with clarity, intelligence or sincerity, it speaks from fear of the unknown. This voice lacks awareness, and plays with our conscious mind. Be mindful about what you think, because you could be defeating how you think if you don't listen and learn from your inner voice speaking to you.

This contradictory inner voice is of negative nature, and it is very illusive in its nature of thinking. This inner voice can push you to make stupid decisions, whether it is in love or at work. This inner voice contradicts your reasonable thoughts. It contradicts and changes the frequency of your thoughts. Then it takes your secret weapons, your determination, your motivation, and your drive to succeed, and controls all your decisions based on your weakness. This is where you need some spiritual secret ammunition. You need true mind power to control the way your mind relates to you.

To keep that inner voice silence, you need to listen to your spiritual guide, and connect at a deeper level so you can bypass what is going on inside your confused mind. You may be saying, "Easier say than done." If you want to silence the thoughts to the voice in your head. You first have to ask your- self, "What am I thinking? Why? How will this help me? Understand the nature of your thought. Figure out where exactly the thoughts are coming from and then, reevaluate them. You may have to go deep inside your conscious mind and connect to your inner spiritual core to get the answers. It is the best way I know how.

People are constantly looking for answers and questions with a purpose. Ask yourself "What do I want?" We are constantly thinking, but our thoughts are not always of good nature. Sometimes, they force themselves into our rational minds and combat our good thought and intentions. Thinking is a process we can control. If we recognize the nature of a thoughts, we can avoid the poison it may bring to our energies, and our minds. Yes, thoughts do have energy; They have the power to control our minds, our conscious, and our physical as well as emotional well-being.

Our conscious and subconscious minds are a constant force of unparalleled power, one is always trying to suppress the other with negative thinking. You have to find the balance between the two and maintain clarity in thinking.

You can lower the frequency of your thoughts. Pick something you like, develop it, work hard on it, and make it happen. Purpose is that which makes us happy, brings us joy, and allow us to share it with others. Purpose increases the frequency of your thoughts and helps you get what you want. To achieve success, you must be aligned with your divine nature, your mind and your heart, together they are the guide to creating miracles in your life. Together they work in harmony to bring joy, and fulfillment. This is how you manifest everything you want. When you are connected to your divine nature, you have found inner peace and wisdom with a profound certainty of who you are. "The mind of God." These **high levels of mind frequency** will take you to unlimited places in your life journey.

Now that you have connected internally, your vision is entirely in your hands. Your conscious and subconscious resources will help you be aware of where you are at all times. The two minds, subconscious, and conscious will no longer battle for control. You have now managed to take control over the conflict that was preventing you from obtaining your goals. You obtained success because you aligned your mind with these wonderful mind techniques. This is not the law of manifestation, where everything happens instantaneously; you have to do the groundwork and set the foundation for what you are about to receive. Nothing comes from magic. Reality is based on your understanding and experiences you process as the events are evolving before you.

YOUR BELIEFS

Putting your thoughts on paper helps you analyze and understand different perspectives about what you want and believe. Writing it on paper helps you manifest what you desire. When you imagine something, you have a mental image; when you to make it a reality because you believed in it. In your ability to manifest what you want. Your beliefs are your perceptions of what you, imagine it to be. Beliefs originate at a conscious level of the mind. Your conviction of your beliefs determines whether you succeed or fail, because you have to have a deep conviction about what you perceive to be real. Your beliefs are created as a child. You then continue to build your beliefs because of what you have learned. What you perceive, and accept, are part of your beliefs, so is what you think.

Be aware about what you are thinking. Making decisions required focus and choices. When in doubt, ask your self, am I making the right decision, or do I need more time to think about it? Always create a balance between your choices of yes and no. Find a happy medium in making the correct choices, but also ask what are the pros- and cons- of your choices. Seek understanding about what is it that you belief. You can believe in yourself or others, the results are always the same. In the end, it is about your connection and your concept about what you belief. Something moves you!

SUCCESS

Success depends on your inner drive to never give up, or your desire to want something bad! Also, it is the persistence of your efforts to get you where you want to go. Our success is like a magnetic field, we acquired it with an inner drive, then work consistently on it, until we have perfected the ideal expression of what we have created in our mind. To be successful, one must also embrace the failures that comes with it. Not all success have failures, but they do have lessons to teach us. Success means different things to different people. For some, success means having money. For others, success simply means having the power to control others. For still others, it's the ability to share knowledge with people. Whatever your preference is, make it the best you can. We cannot all live by the same standards. Success for me is the gratification of having achieved something that I can share with others. Life to me is about sharing my gift with others. Only then, can I receive all the blessings I deserve.

VISUALIZATION

What we see, we perceive, what we perceive, we will believe, visualize, and then we make it happen. Then it manifest in our life's. Visualization is like a child's imagination. The reality of it is so vivid that the child actually believes it to be true. This is the same way we have to visualize what we want in life. The experience of visualization is so creative, that we can actually live in a world of our own making. Visualization is the vivid experience of our incredible ability to imagine things even though they are not there. Before you can make something come to life, you must first imagine it as if it was real. You can even have feelings when you have imagined something in your mind. You can live it, feel it, sense it, and believe that is true. That is the powerful influence of a creative mind. This creative imagination is the reason why many inventions and new ideas become reality. To visualize something, you must see your future beyond the now. Use your creative mind to make your dreams a reality.

TAKE ACTION

Once you have created and idea, visualized it, and seen it alive in your life, then you can take action. Don't simply create an idea and let it flow. Put it on paper, and imagine how it will feel. Vividly live the moment and then, project that idea into the universe. You have to do what you say you will do. See yourself as the creator of the idea. Take credit for something when you have taken action. Taking action means that you have made a step into acting upon your desire dream. Now, you should let go of the anticipation and allow the universe to take over for you. What this means is that you let go without hesitation and have faith in what you have done. You, the inventor of the idea have already put sufficient energy to let it manifest into your life. Now, it is all about the law of the universe to make it happen for you. We can't control all outcome; taking action is the first step one can make, then with our energy and vibration will allow it to happen.

CORRECT YOUR MISTAKES TO BALANCE YOUR MIND

You must be wondering, *"How in the world, can I correct the past errors in my life?"*

Mistakes are errors we made as a result of poor judgment or choices. Such as a career, abortion, marrying the wrong person for the wrong reasons, and so on. To make a transition from wrong to right,you have to analyze what you did, understand it, apologize if you have to, forgive, and forget, make the changes, and move on.

The best example I can give you is a relationship between two people. You meet your future partner, you get engage, you both live together for a while before setting the wedding day. But your expectations of this person are not what you had imagined. You realized that you had made a mistake. How do you break the news to your partner without hurting his or her feelings. No matter the outcome of this situation, you are both going to be hurt and experience from it. There is no sweet way about it. Now that you know you have made a mistake, you explain, forgive yourself, accept it, understand the other persons feelings, respect, and let it go, you move on. This is the best way to solve and correct the mistake, heal your mind, so you can move on without pain or guilt. Correction of any kind is the ability to put into practice now what you have learned and experienced in the past.

Correcting your past mistakes is how your thoughts can help you balance from within. You learn to make a difference in your life with all the situations you have previously encountered. You are constantly learning from your past mistakes; it is a way to grow. The more you understand about how to correct your past mistakes, the faster you will move forward and deal with life in a more profound prudent manner. You will learn that if you have hurt someone in the past, now have the power to forgive yourself and ask for forgiveness, you can learn, move on and grow. It is all about having empathy for others. This is also a healthy way of releasing yourself from guilt. Everything that you do and plan in life begins with a thought. Think healthy and move on with your life. We cannot escape the mind's ability to be multifunctional and flexible, at the same time, but we can transform how we use our mind. If you ever heard people say they are not able to change their habits or mistakes; that is wrong! They simply don't want to. They can do so, if their minds are in accord with their well-being. Whatever the case is, there is hope. We can all correct what we have done wrong. Even in the worst of cases, the power to make up for wrong-doing in the past is in our minds. We are more mentally capable than we recognize.

BE STILL

The Bible says, "Be still and know that I am." This is a very important message. When you are still, you can feel a sense of peace, a sense of oneness with who you are, you can connect with your inner self. Being still means to be at peace with the self for a moment. In stillness, you find answers, you get to know who you are, and you connect to levels of your mind you haven't experienced before. You can listen to that inner voice of reason that talks to you when you need it. You will have more clarity in your thinking when you are silent.

Stillness is a privilege we don't often have because we don't take advantage of it. We are constantly busy with our thoughts. If you don't know how to experience stillness, you will not discover your ability to learn to listen to your inner voice. It is important that we listen to ourselves internally to be able to express externally how we truly feel. We live in a world of high demands; our ability to connect to our inner world is limited by our lifestyle. But for those who are conscious enough to connect through meditation, the results are creativity, and the capacity to react and think with awareness. Life is more than we experience on a daily basis. We are limited by nothing but separation from our ability to think clearly. With stillness, we are able to see beyond the now.

In stillness, you open the portal of an unknown creation thus becoming more attune with yourself. Stillness uplift your inner spirit to connect you to something greater or unimaginable more powerful than you. Be still and know thyself. Stillness is inner tranquility; it is the gift of life that keeps giving us more understanding, more knowledge, and more wisdom. It is a feeling of connection with all that we are. You are not what the world presents, rather, you are what you find within you. Your deepest conscious understanding and true nature of your gift. You are part of all stillness. Remain still; experience peace, calmness, love, space, and find the answers to all your unknown questions. Don't get lost or cut up into all the things of this world. Find time for you to be still and be one with yourself. You are in the universe and of the universe. Be still and know that you are.

BE WILLING

Willingness gives you courage and the strength necessary to change. The willpower of life is a willingness to continue living. When you thrive, you are willing to succeed to make a transition, and you have found the willpower to want to change. In order for us to succeed, we have to want to make a difference in this world, or else, there is no purpose for success. When you are willing to change or make a difference in this world, you must also face the reality and struggles of what it means to succeed. Many people struggled to succeed, but only those who are willing to be uncomfortable do make it. Willingness is spontaneity and vulnerability at the same time.

Willingness is an inner drive, a willpower that pushes you when you are ready to go beyond where you are now. When you are willing, you think about how to make a difference to transform your life and improve your chances for a better future. To be willing means that you are ready to make a shift; you are able to take chances, and you have handed yourself over to the opportune time to make things happen. Willingness in itself is transformation. In willingness, you surrender to the outcome of all or any possibility coming into your life for the choices you make. You are not concern about the outcome but you allow the expression of that outcome to flow with you. When I surrender all to God, I am letting go of the things that can hold me back, thus I create space for the good things to come. In willingness there is no resistance, all things flow through me voluntarily.

SEEK BEYOND THE NOW

Be curious about your life, and your imagination, where you want to go, how you want to get there, and what steps you are willing to take to make it happen. See beyond the now. Creative imagination is greater than knowledge. If you are able to create ideas, you can create the future, make a difference and reach beyond the borders of the unknown. Seeking beyond the present means you are able to take you mind deep into the unknown were only great geniuses have gone before; you go where others have not gone before.

Many great inventors of our time had a creative mind; they had a drive that was never satiated, a mind that did not stop thinking, or generating new ideas until they found what they were seeking. That is how you seek beyond where you are, to where you want to go, you continue to try to find the answers for the things you believe to be true.

You ask questions, make your own assumptions, and create your conclusions in accordance to your knowledge of the facts. You don't just get stuck in the now and hope to find the answers, you go looking for them. You dare yourself to go where others have not gone before. You challenge your mind to think, calculate, and rationalize all your questions. Eventually, you will find the answers. Seek, look, think, know and understand about the things that bring curiosity into your mind and you shall find them. Don't ever make assumptions without knowing the fact, seek for true knowledge. Knowledge is wisdom and wisdom is power. Internal power generates a force that when seeking for the unknown or the truth is unstoppable!

THE POWER WITHIN

Life sometimes throws situations at us that forces us to make drastic and quick decisions for survival. Some refer to this as survival mode, which means fear or fight is when you are confronted with a life or death situation. Your decision to make the right choice is within your power. Whether you believe it or not, we all have this power in us.

Trust in yourself and know that you can. When your anxious thoughts multiply within you, but know that your hope delights in your spirit. You are powerful! Trust in yourself and know that you can. There are times when people freeze and are unable to respond. This means they don't act well under pressure. They cannot make rational, concise decisions to save themselves.

Imagine that you are the only person well enough to fly an airplane, but you don't have any previous flying experience. Would you take the wheel and try to do your best or would you let everyone die? This type of thinking gives you the ability to think with your inner power, and make a rational decision. The voice within your mind will speak for you. You will know what to do unless you are the type of person who cannot react or think rationally under severe pressure. You will be amazed at how quickly people respond in a moment like this, reaction kicks in and survival mode is in gear. The norm is that most people will do the best they can under pressure. That is the power we possess within us. This power within is similar to the animal instinct. When an animal is hunting, it sees, it aims, it measures distance and perimeters, then it goes, it attacks its target. We are not different, except we do it with our human instincts or intuition, our gut feelings.

KNOW THYSELF

Do you have dreams and desires you want to achieve in your life? Do you want to know who you are? Do you believe you are the remnants of the big bang? or are you the creation of God's imagination, an imagination that began with thoughts. Who are you? A human being. Are you part of the dust from a supernova with gamma rays that burst atoms into the universe with neutrinos? Neutrinos are the particles that makes up the building blocks of life. So, again, who are you? Are you a soul, a spirit, a conscious mind, or the consciousness of your thoughts? We are all spirited beings with souls, with energy, with purpose, and with a conscious mind that help us function in life. But who you are has to do with your dream, your purpose, your fulfillments or your spirited being. You are a soul with energy guided by that which created you. What you are is hidden in you within your subconscious mind. To know thyself requires that you open up completely, and expose yourself to know you, the person, the feelings, the emotional intelligence, your faults, your fears, your joy, your happiness, your sadness, and all that is you. Again, I ask, who are you? Are you a light that permeates throughout the universe?

You are a loving soul! That is what you are. Stop searching for you. You are here. Know who you are. We are not the things that make us, we are that which we are. The word universe means all, that indeed we are. If we exist, then we are part of all existence.

FAITH AND TRANSFORMATION

To have faith is to believe, to transcend beyond the now, to choose to connect to something greater than yourself. At some point in our life,we all believe in something outside ourselves. Something that connected us to a higher level of spiritual experience to what we normally know or think we know. We cannot have faith nor believe unless we have pure thoughts and a deep conviction about what is it that we believe in. Faith creates a foundation for something to guide us into a higher spiritual connection to a divine force outside ourselves. Think of faith as a GPS, it is guiding you to a designated place, while lack of it is getting you lost into the unknown. We should avoid limitations within our convictions and depend on something with a greater power than our own. Otherwise, we would not need changes or transformation. We would be perfect human beings. Adam and Eve brought consciousness into existence with their knowledge by recognizing their sins. The fact that they knew they were naked, help them become conscious about it. Before that, they knew not about their naked bodies. We, human beings do not recognize faith until it is experience from a need to have faith. Sometimes, a life trauma, a lost of a loved one, or a near death experienced can awaken faith in us. Faith is born in the heart, not found outside of us. Faith creates spiritual as well as emotional balance, and we all need it to transform our mind. We need peace of mind, knowledge, joy, and a connection to something that helps us understand what we don't understand. Without faith we could not put a name to what happens when we experience something we don't understand.

We all have different preferences when it comes to beliefs. I am not trying to instill a religious belief or change your perception about your religion; rather, I am trying to connect the experience one shares when connecting to a divine or greater power. I understand that not everyone sympathizes with my view, and that is okay with me. Faith can be described in many facets: Either you have it or you experience it through others. It is all up to you, the individual. I do know that for me, and my personal experiences, there is a meaning that I cannot put into words. I have been able to connect all my experiences, and what I have learned in life with my faith to know what faith means to me. Thus, I conclude that without it, I wouldn't have being here today to write these pages of my book. It was in a moment of desperation when I experienced sadness, despair and pain that faith saved me. I tried to do it alone, but somehow I felt. I need something greater than I to help me from my lost and spiritual anguish. I will not be insulted if you don't share my opinion. Tragically, if you don't have faith to move forward in life, then you will experience conflict and negative experiences. Trying to do things on your own never works. No matter who you are or how strong your convictions are, there is a power outside ourselves which guides us in this incredible universe we live in. Whether it is your self- awareness about God in you, or your divine power as inherited knowledge of the mind of God, there is something! Trying to have faith without a pure conviction about something is like navigating a new route without a GPS. You will get lost. Transformation of the mind without faith cannot happen. You will have a difficult time allowing progress to come to you. Nonetheless, the transformation of your thoughts will not happen. You will constantly fight with your inner conflicts. Faith is more powerful when practiced, but it can have a greater effect in your life if you strongly believe.

When you have faith or belief, you are calm, relax in your own state of being with your mind at ease. You are no preoccupied with unnecessary mundane things. Life seems to have meaning and more value because you are in peace with yourself. Something has brought that peace to you, your faith in it. As you connect to your source or what you know, you tap into the level of your conscious mind that helps you experience a new state of consciousness and communication with an alter state of being you didn't know you had. When you believe, you place no limitations upon your thoughts or your desires, rather you move forward with faith and certainty in what you want. You can see all that was hidden with clarity. Your mental empowerment is but your perception about your belief and how you feel about it. You understand that what is guiding this universe is much more powerful than you. That in itself is enough to believe.

Faith is like the cosmological forces of the universe: the more we believe, the more we attract and experience all that is. Belief gives us energy in a positive direction in order to gain momentum and reach our goals. Something we don't precisely know has a hold on our spiritual being. If you believe in nothing, then you have nothing to lean on.

We understand that 75% percent of the universe is occupied by dark energy. Dark energy is a force that dominates the universe's four forces and causes the universe to expand.

Likewise, beliefs, thoughts, and a unified collection of thoughts do have an impact upon us and the rest of the world. What you think can affects the people around you. It also affects natural forces of the universe. Faith is energy, a powerful voltage that charges our spirits, our minds, our bodies, and everything that moves us forward. Faith gives us mind power, and spiritual power, a force inside our deepest conscious level that helps us think, and act in a compassionate manner with others. Faith is the primordial force of spiritual power that gives you the empathy to forgive, love and care for others. Without it, we would not forgive or accept judgment, resentment, and hate. You can overcome all with faith. You have to believe in order to let go of that which you have no power to control.

In moments of desperation, we all turn to God, and our thoughts lean on him. We look for him to help us find the answers to some of the most painful and doubtful moments in our life. When we feel powerless, or our mind is in turmoil, we turn to him for help. If you ever reach a level of desperation in life where you needed an answer to make a difficult decision, who did you ask for help? I know that some of us could not do it alone. You surrender your life when you are powerless, and you let go and let him guide you. You ask and you receive. Remember that in faith you are empower, you are confident in yourself and others, you have a deep trust in you and what is guiding you throughout your life. Faith is transformation from within. However, we cannot explain faith in its entirety, one must experience it to understand its true meaning in their life. In faith all things are possible.

When you finally get your prayers answered, that's when you really know is your faith at work. When you are able to turn to him, this is when you begin to use the power of positive thinking. You begin to use the power of positive thinking. Faith is an integral part of our life. If you surrender your power to him, you will begin to discover peace of mind. Then you will know that no matter what, all is well. In silence you will find confidence, his power, and your willingness to find strength where before you were weak. You direct everything to the power of your mind and will find yourself in God consciousness. Know that consciousness is the ultimate mind awareness or tool to finding spiritual power. This consciousness is how we connect to the unknown, is where we become aware and relate to it without seeing it. Ask yourself, can a conscious mind commit a crime? Not very likely, for when you do any of these, you are not conscious of who you are. There is no consciousness in wrong-doing, in that state, you are either unconscious or acting upon your subconscious domain. A conscious mind is aware of its actions, thoughts, reactions and doing. It cannot act without the consent of a rational logical mind.

THINK POSITIVE AND DEFEAT FEAR

When your life is moving forward, you know that you are in the right place, at the right time. You are here because you have made the right changes in your life to get you where you are.

Now, think positive and know that you have something to offer to someone, somewhere in the world. Someone is waiting to hear these words to feel better, to change their life, or to make a change that could transform how they think. Someone is looking for what exactly you have to offer. To understand your gift, you have to know what motivates you. What drives you inside, and what gives you fulfillment in life? These are the questions you should be asking yourself. Dare to do what you love without fear. Those who fear neglect themselves from the challenges that can bring them satisfaction, prosperity and fulfillment in life.

Don't be anxious or stress about what you want in life. To get what you want, you must live life with passion. Seek and set your goals because they will manifest from your deepest desires. Remember that your journey in life requires effort, dedication, discipline, and the determination to make it happen. Your capacity to make things happen is effortless, however how you try to make it happen does make difference. Positive or negative thoughts influence the outcome of everything you want and plan in your life. Think positively and, allow your mind to help you manifest your desires. Your ability to think is knowledge, which is empowerment and creates growth. Knowledge is a way of obtaining power. Thinking positive defeats fear which is created in your subconscious mind because it wants to avoid confrontation. Have no fear, and empower your mind to think positively. All positive power comes from within and is under your control.

Fear and negative thinking are both the results of a powerless feeling or an inability to achieve your goals because of influential thinking. This thought mechanism makes you doubt yourself, thus creates fear in you. Think positively, believe in yourself, and let go of control. Believe in your own mental power, which conquers anything you want. The power of your thoughts carries a magnetic field that reflects internally as well as externally; this is how you reveal yourself to the outside world. Know that your thoughts carry energy and vibration with them which makes them manifest in your life. Think positively and attract all the magnetism and positive energy that is around you with the power of your mind. Your thoughts magnetic field spread all the way to universe and back. This is how one idea can enter the mind of multiple people at the same time; this idea is in the field of everything, and those who tune in with their mind can grasp at it. Positive thinking requires no efforts only that you focus with your mind.

Thoughts carry a powerful force. With your thoughts, you can create war, hate, or love. Your thoughts can influence others, you, and everything that comes to and develops around you. Watch what you are thinking. Trust and listen to your thoughts because they have unlimited power. Use them in a constructive manner. With your thoughts, you can think yourself into success or failure, you choose. They serve as an autosuggestion to our mind. They drive us, direct us, control us, make us feel or not, and they can create what is and is not there. Example: You can put yourself into a depression by thinking about something negative or a past painful experience. You can be happy by feeling emotions that once made you feel good, joyful and happy. The mind is like a switch, you can turn it on happy or turn it on sad; the results are up to you. We have the power of our mind in our hands, just like that! Pay attention to what comes into your mind. To overcome the pattern of negative thinking, simply replace the negative thoughts with an autosuggestion that says, "Not now! You don't need negative vibrations in your life. Keep it simple. Don't overpower your mind with your thoughts. Your thoughts can be constructive or not; you decide. Control your mind to think constructively rather than self-destructively. If you do it without hesitation, you will have constant effectiveness. Withdraw your mind from the negative habits of your past and commit yourself 100 percent.

The power is in you. The power of positive thinking is so magical and effective that it only takes one change in your perception, then the momentum begins. Plus you put into practice what you have learned to stay aware and positive. Dominate the power of your inner voice, your thoughts, then you will find out who you really are, fearless. Remember that the voice you will hear the most is your own voice. Restrain your thinking, build confidence, and limit your beliefs to create a healthy mind. And find out who you really are, fearless.

Many scientists asks who we are and from where we come? Why are we here? Why do we think, speak or evolve? Why are we smarter than our predecessors? How did we evolve from the caveman to a new creature of intelligence? Who we are is an entire evolution and transition of language and thinking. We are here today because of our a primordial efforts to survive each predecessors and climatic changes along the path. Who we are is a puzzling question in the minds of doubters. Nonetheless, who we are is conscious powerful spirited human beings with an insatiable and limitless capacity to create with our mind. We are unlike no other creatures in the universe.

We are the purpose of our lives, we are the creation of a new idea that began with a thought. Once you understand how significant you are in this universe, then you know that you are part of all that exists. We are part of this universe, therefore, you are the creation of all that exists within the realms of space and time. We were created with a purpose. In other words, you are God's purpose and you have a purpose.

If you want to mastermind all aspects of your life, let go of your fears, be honest with yourself, then get in the habit of knowing what you want from life. Find your life purpose and discover your goals.

You owe yourself the opportunity to make a change in your life if you are not happy.

Happiness reflects you outwards. There is an internal mirror the world can see in your facial expression reflecting outwards. And it is who you are. Happy or sad, no matter what? Sometimes, the truth can be told without an image or spoken words. Is there. Happiness is within you, and only you can find it. Take a leap of faith, change your thinking, and be happy. Let go of the fear and begin anew. Life is a beautiful journey. My journey began when I expressed myself honestly from the heart. The truth can be told better when it is spoken from the heart.

You have no one to blame for your failures, if you are not honest for the results of their outcome. Or why did you fail? You can practice visualization daily, but unless you change and conform to how you have programmed your subconscious mind with negative thoughts, your positive visualization will not help you. Transformation comes from within, and change is a need for reforming what you are not comfortable with or happy in your life. Growing allows you to reach further than you could possibly imagine. Change is good, it feels good, and gives you a new perspective in life: to maintain your drives and to manifest good things in your life. If you are a person who procrastinates about doing something or finds excuses, then you are not being honest with yourself; You are not listening to your intuition, your inner voice. The messages and words you are speaking are not spoken from your heart. You are not telling the truth. You find alternate excuses to stop yourself from excelling. When you are honest and open with yourself, you are more likely to make progress and excel in life.

When you go against your purpose in life, you will constantly face adversity. Not matter how much effort you put into your future plans, you will find out you cannot win. Then you will have a wake-up call, or an "aha" moment. You will have a need to change. You can go deep inside yourself to seek for answers with your eyes closed and a quite mind. Silence is the best precursor to finding your answers. Sometimes you will cry, pray, ask for guidance, or get on your knees. You will begin to see changes as soon as you stop being anxious about it. You will find peace of mind and comfort once you let go of the anticipations.

Until you have released the fear and the shattering in your mind, you will not see changes. Everything will remain the same. Change happens when you, make the decision to go inward and understand why you are eliciting negative thoughts. When your thinking is affecting the way you feel and your emotional intelligence, it is time to bring back the magic. You must write down what is happening with your emotions, scrutinize it, and believe that you can change the way you feel. You then remove your attention from the bad thoughts because, you cannot have bad and good thoughts at the same time.

This is not about other people's feelings, and this is not about what people think or believe about you. This is about improving the quality of your own life. It is about telling yourself the truth about what is going on inside you. You have to tell it from the heart. You have to be honest to yourself so that you can be happy. You have to be honest to yourself so that you can be happy. If you want to think positive and let go of the fear, you must build a strong mind.

If you want to change the way you think, change the frequency of your thoughts. Believe that what you think, you will attract into your life. Understand how the nature of your thoughts creates your reality. There is a balance in the way we think; good thoughts, good vibrations and good energy. Negative thoughts equals negative energy and vibration. Think differently in order to make a change. Thinking is all about a mindset; it is about the ability to maintain a balance between you, your mind, and what comes to it when you allow it. Control your thoughts, your emotions, and reactions around places and people, train your mind to be aware of your thoughts and commands at all times. Be the operator of your own creative mind. You take control of your mind and your life the way you want. Now that you have power over your own thoughts, there is no more fear. You are the protagonist of your own thoughts.

If you have a tendency to be very critical about people, then you can train your mind to be completely aware. Have compassion instead of being critical. When you have a critical thought, stop it and become aware instantly. Remind yourself not to go there. This is an auto-suggestion sent to your mind for a positive response. Be compassionate and replace sinister criticism. It's that easy to swift the way you think. Beware of your thoughts about yourself and others, and create more compassion with an open heart. Compassion toward others is a kinder act of love that is expressed deeply from the heart. It is a feel-good kind of feeling.

MIND POWER

When you achieve mind power, the rewards are peace of mind and positive thinking, abundance and good things manifest in your life. This is possible because you have recognized the power you have to control your mind. Without this power, you can be manipulated by the people around you. Here is a good example: Today's society is geard towards manipulating our minds with images, and messages to influence the public to buy what they sell. Sex is another form of creative manipulation which is use to influence a buyers mind. There are many forms of mind control and deception going on today. You must build a tough mind not to be influenced nor controlled by others. Let me make it more simple; throughout history, society, and the rich influencer have suppressed minorities, we all know this. However as our evolution progress continues, we become more consciously aware of our mental capacity and what is evolving all around us. We are not longer ignorant sentient beings, but we have learned the importance of our mental power. Now, the message is clear for those who try so desperately to coarse and control our minds; our intellectual cognitive abilities are no different than theirs, we are the new conscious awaken generation. Change is like a magnet: one can only attract what one is thinking. Once you have recognize who you are as a human being, your strength and confidence with your mental power begins to grow. You are not longer under the control nor manipulated by others, rather you are in complete control of your life.

If you want to overcome your powerlessness, take the time to do the things you like, rather than being influenced by what others do or why. To become mentally strong you have to work at building you up instead of handing over your power to others. It is normal to feel powerless or broken inside before you regain your power; In your brokenness, there is also power. Vulnerability is surrendering the old to give birth to something new. If you want to recognize the power of your mind, challenge yourself do something you always fear doing. Mental power is a transformation of the mind from uncertainty and doubts to a total control of your full mental capacity.

TRUE-SELF

We often doubt and ask ourselves questions that only we know the answers to. The true self can be found with the law of connection, via synchronicity. This law binds all things together. You can go from having nothing to having happiness and fulfillment. But you must ask yourself, "What keeps me from being my true self?" When we don't listen to our intuition or gut feelings, we create uncertainty where there is none. Doubt and uncertainty are one and the same. We doubt because we are not certain; and we are certain because we do not doubt. But if we listen to our inner voice, there is never doubt nor uncertainty in our choices or questions. Sometimes, when you have any confrontation with the external world is because you have to deal with some unsolved internal issues. The external is an expression of our inner complex conflicts. Often time we forget that the most important thing in our life is to know thyself. We have a tendency to want to work on solving other people's problems instead of our own. When you take the time and efforts to re-evaluate who you are, you will find out how often you neglect yourself to give to others. To know yourself is to be wide open with yourself about who you are, what moves you, what makes you happy or unhappy. To know you is to love you, to be authentic with thoughts, feelings, emotions, and hiding nothing from you.

Authenticity and self-love is found when you create the time to value who you are and nourish the child within; that child who is always seeking and asking for more self- love.

If you ever felt that there was more to life than were you were in that moment, then you needed to make a change. The fact that you ask tells you that you are not satisfy where you are. Perhaps, because you were not honest with yourself, you had to ask. The best way to know yourself is to be honest. Honesty, like integrity are important to express your true self. Being honest means that you listen to your inner voice, and you make decisions based on your own cognitive intelligence of it. To create an authentic expression of who you are, you need to be you, do you, and express who you are without hesitation. To accomplish this, it is essential that you work on the things you want to change and build a new you. Remember, no one can do for you what you can do for yourself. Self-fulfillment and accomplishment are your sole efforts, but the rewards are pure transformation and self-love. Self-love is to know thyself. To know you is to trust you; to have mind power you must to be authentic with yourself.

True self-discovery comes from within, not from the external world. If you manage to do it yourself, you will truly change and achieve remarkable success. This transformation will enhance your experience for life. You will feel the inner sensation that something greater than you has taken over and manifested inside you. Allow yourself to evolve, and pursue new horizons to help you expand your mind.

When you consistently relate to the past in the present, you have begun to loose your mind power. Consequently, you begin to lose yourself. True mind power is conceived when you are present in the moment, thus you are aware of your full mind control. When we say we have mind power, it means that we control our emotions and our thoughts when people push our boundaries. It also means that we are capable of handling whatever comes our way without loosing control of our rational thinking. Therefore, one can always remain calm to deal diligently with anything happening outside which is out of one's control. Strength doesn't affect our emotional well-being. We can be sensitive and be strong at the same time.

We all posses a strong mind, but we don't always use the power of our mind to our advantage.

If there is one time when we are challenged with the power of our mind is when we have lost a loved one. In this instance, we also loose part of our true self. We become sad, weak, cry, and there is a deep feeling of lost in our soul.

Why is it so difficult to let go and move on? Why do we lose control of our feelings and emotions when someone passes on? We know we are all going to die, sometime.

Death is one of those moments when we cannot control ourselves, we loose our ability to mend our emotions back together. It seems to take a long time to get over the grief and sadness. Nonetheless in this moment when we are being so vulnerable, we are our true authentic self.

But regardless of who you are or what has happened, you will tend to loose your rational thinking mind as you linger into deep sadness until you learn to let it go!

When we surrender, we are being honest with ourselves. Being true to yourself requires you to be weak before you become strong.

There are times in our lives when we are powerless, thus in those moments we cannot reason why we feel a certain way, we simply know that it happens to some of us.

Although our behavior tells the world how we feel, what we think about the world and our concept about reality, there is not doubt that sometimes our thoughts can be affected by the environment. Have you ever heard the expression "actions speak louder than words".

Well, that is so true. Our actions are the influence by the energy of our thoughts. When we think about something, there is an energy invisible by nature that propels those thoughts into a higher frequency to make us act or react. Some people may refer to this as emotions, or impulses. Anyways,

I believe that they are like the neutrinos in the atmosphere, which are invisible but powerful enough to feel the mind with energy. A neutrino is a subatomic particle that have no electrical charges but travel at near light speed. If you want to know yourself better, write down ten things positive that you like about yourself. Think about the last time you did something that brought you joy, happiness , but you had to work very hard at creating this thing. What was the feeling, how did you celebrate the accomplishment of it? Now, think about something you try to do but you failed at making it happen. What was it that cause you to fail, why did you stop, what was the end result, and how did you feel? Now that you know the end results of your failures and accomplishments; you acknowledge them by being honest with yourself. This is what it means to Know thyself.

"Speak thou thy truth, allow thy honesty to flourish through thy thoughts, thy mind will proclaim who thou are, and thy thoughts will become healthier with time".

GOOD HABITS

If you believe that putting your thoughts into action is difficult, then you are denying yourself the ability to grow. Awareness takes seconds; habits take a lifetime. Shifting is an immediate choice. To put your thoughts into actions is a determination. Change is an instant action, and a manifestation of your innermost desires. Good habits are cultivated with your mind's ability to differentiate between positive or negative thoughts. To manifest the power of your thoughts, you have to know where your mind is going, what you are thinking, and why have you generated these thoughts. The miraculous power of the mind is that it has the ability to take you anywhere you want to go. Your mind has the ability to take you into the past and bring you back. It can also take you into the future. All you have to do is imagine!

Your mind reactivates these thoughts whenever you ask it to do so. Good habits are those that, although they are part of the past, will bring you pleasure and fulfillment in the present. They are connected to the happy moments of your memories. They are part of what makes you, you!

Bad habits will brake you and destroy your ability to think rationally. Your thoughts are a pyramid that builds up only as long as you, the thinker continues to contribute to the vibration of your thoughts.

Don't let your habitual mind judge the value of your thoughts. Use your intelligence to practice what you have learned, then allow your knowledge, and understanding to bring you joy with fulfillment. We all have a gift to share with the world, but our habits not always help us develop this gift. Don't let your bad habits rob you of your gifts. Create good habits that elevate your imagination and help you fulfill your desires. Good habits contribute to greater imagination. Miracles happen to those who believe in themselves, their inner voices, and their intuitions. Use your good habits to help you improve your knowledge, intelligence and achieve your goals to help you feel joy and fulfillment in life.

Your creative imagination will keep you growing, and your ideas will flourish with time. The greater the disciple and efforts you put into it, the greater the end results. Good habits with motivation are the two driving forces that pushes us to prove what we are made of. Without motivation, we loose momentum, then getting it back becomes a struggle. With good habits comes dedication; dedication creates enthusiasm to finish what we star. On the contrary, bad habits can destroyed our dreams, contribute to our laziness, and make us fail when we should have succeed. Let not your bad habits destroy your dreams. They will must certainly show up with you at your burial site. You can discover the genius in you. Geniuses are not made, they are created. When you have tried to do your best in life, you can discover the genius in you. Our thoughts create all, and so talent can be learned. Consistency and routine are the results of today's greatest inventions and imagination. Everything that was ever created came from the imagination and intelligence of men and women who created good habits to help them achieve their goals. The values of your thoughts will determine all that you dream and want in your life. But remember, it takes self-discipline and commitment to get what you want.

It takes dedication to make any improvements in life. It is my expereince as a writer that once I have created the habit of writing at a dedicated time everyday of the week, I will continue with my dedication and persistence until I am done. Good habits are the end results of creating a good schedule to follow without falling back on a project. It does help you accoplish your task, and helps you build your trust. Yes, you can trust yourself to finish what you started, be present, and get it done!

Your job becomes a habit with time, but before you can fully master your job, you have to learn to create discipline and a good habit to work with. Otherwise, you will be all over the place without making progress. Everyhting that we do in life rquires decipline and good habits.

As the saying goes, bad habits are hard to break. It takes disciple to want to change the way you are used to doing what you do. This old way of doing things is like an addiction, you have to get rid of it, if you want to improve how you function mentally. To change your habits, you have to train your mind to want to think differently, then invasion a new perspective about how you want to accomplish this. However, your desires will be the driving force that helps you do it.

Chapter 5

Awareness Will Expand Your Mind

IF YOU ASK YOURSELF THE following questions you will create space to
Create space to expand your mind
What are your habits?
What are you attached to?
When and how you change how you think now?
How would you benefit from these changes?

Knowing what you want is important for you to have a clear vision.

When we are open minded we do not resist changes, rather change happen because we are willing and able to receive them without resistance.

Remember that negative thinking resists change. Focus on your intent and discipline yourself to work on these efforts every day until you, have achieved success. But most importantly, do not resist change. Once you remove all habits, good things will follow. Remember to celebrate every effort that you make to change. Rewards are good ways to give yourself a gift of gratitude. Awareness is key because you can release old habits, build new patterns of behavior, think clear, and build a better mental state. You no longer operate under the commands of your weak mind, the unconscious mind. You, the person who once had habits and a weak mind, can now control your thoughts and all outcomes.

Your bad habits can deprive you from self-awareness thus impede your possibilities to expand your mind beyond the now. Without awareness, you are stock in the moment, and you cannot make progress. Awareness is how wild animals in the kingdom recognize danger and act quickly away from predators. Your awareness is your alarm system, when you expand your awareness with your mind, you embodied certainty no doubt. Wake up every day with a desire to do something you love and enjoy completely. Be aware of what makes you happy and enjoy everything life has to offer you as you become more aware of yourself and others.

Every day brings a new opportunity for you to improve, to listen, and to understand who you are. As you go through the day, remind yourself who you are, why you are here, and what you want to obtain for yourself. What do you have to offer to the world, to you and to other people? By examining where you are and comparing it to where you want to be, you are making a step forward into creating your personal goals.

Life doesn't end because we stop aim for our goals, there is always time standing waiting for us to be aware of our mind expansion. It is never too late. There is a constant motion that moves with the internal energy you send out into the universe. What energy are you sending out into the universe today? Recognize and allow your emotions to flow through as you replace old habits with new ones and create a new state of mind. Your mind is the best alarm system you have. It will alert you when you are in danger, let you know when you are wrong, create space for more mistakes, and critique you when you feel bad about yourself, then bring you back to your sanity. But if you allow your mind to become self-aware, it will build expansion for you to grow. As you advance into the process of understanding your new state of mind, you have entered into a state of expansion between you, your mind, and your thought control. This can be considered mastering the old mind and controlling your life outcome with awareness. What a great ability the mind has! In any progress you wish to make in life, awareness is essential. Without awareness, you cannot recognize the problem or the cause of it. Without awareness, you cannot make sense of all that happens internally or externally. Life is a constant learning experience, in the process we create perfections and imperfections, thus we become aware of who or what we are-an imperfect human being.

Expansion is growing from the inside out and learning to recognize who we are in the process.

Sometimes digging deep to find our true character and our passion requires much self-awareness. To be inspire with our dreams and our goals, we have to go beyond the essence of what moves us and touches our deep core. Find your true passion in life, and you will find ultimate happiness. Find out what motivates you? Sometimes your thoughts will deceive you, but most of the time they will lead you into the path of happiness, and fulfillment. Learn to distinguish confusing thoughts from creative ones. Life is meant to be happy. Don't give in to negative thinking, create healthy thoughts. Beware of yourself and create space for an ultimate life experience with your mind expansion that would take you into an unlimited path of possibilities. Let your mind guide you to create treasures with your imagination.

These experiences are worth every learning steps. The pursuit of happiness can transform your life because it will prepare you completely to enjoy the gifts and benefits life has to offer you. Nothing is more rewarding than having the power to deal with all that comes your way. Throughout our life time, when in pursue of our purpose, we may cross many paths with unforgettable memorable experiences learned as tools to help us guide others. Your challenges and learning lessons can only serve as a tool and consolation with loving support to those in similar situations. In the here and now, you begin to understand that your gift is but a perfect pursuit to make others happy, because this journey is not about you. Everything in life is useful; nothing is wasted. When you think that your life is total chaos without outcome or meaning, remember that your lessons are the uplifting gift you can give and share to other people in need to transform their lives from turmoil to happiness.

The only true pursuit of happiness I ever known is to share my gift with others. When life throws a punch you don't see it coming. It is difficult to cope with emotional confrontations and conflicts, but your ability to deal with it will make you a more self-reliable individual. The only perfection we need in life is to learn to control and master our emotions. Thereafter, we can control our mind, our thoughts and our reactions with conscious awareness. After the death of my father, faced with a divorce, and the recollection of the death of my three newborn years past, I felt lost emotionally. I was at the burg of a nervous breakdown. I felt as if I was loosing my mind. I was angry, sad, depress, lonely, and without consolation. I had no one to mourn with. I was away from home without much emotional support. My mind got the best of me. Emotionally, I was a train rack about to crash. If you have never face multiple emotional experiences at the same time, you would never understand what was going on through my mind. I was angry at myself, my ex-husband, my family because I couldn't be present when my father die, plus I was angry at the entire world for not understanding how I was feeling. Unaware of my behavior, I started to write and express myself with words. But these words were not enough. I cry, I dance, I fasted, I experienced many sleepless nights. I was going through so...many emotions at the same time, that I didn't know how to pull myself back to normal. Eventually, I had an aha moment I had decided to attend a meditation class. It was here that I begun to expand my inner spiritual self to gain some peace of mind.

Self-awareness is the byproduct of self-consciousness, but no one is ever fully self-aware when one is too comfortable in life. Because one is never prepared enough for life's outcome, at 61 years old, I was nor ready to start my life anew. I had planned to stay married until I die. Then my life took a 360 degree turn. It wasn't lack of awareness rather, it was an unexpected surprise I felt when life threw a punch at me. I was being tested. I had a wake up call. Though the emotional experience felt as if my world had ended, If I had still be married today, I wouldn't have the beautiful lessons life has taught me. Furthermore, even though I was aware of myself, I wasn't consciously tune into to my true gifts. My life felt as if it had being wasted away without being fulfilled. I had a dream and that dream was dying inside of me. There are many stories barred beneath the ground, My story wasn't about to be one to them. When I was thirteen years old, I had a premonition that one day, I was going to be a very important person in my life. But as the years went by, I lost that dream. That dream was melting away with my age in time. I came to the conclusion that my learned habits were sabotaging my future and my dreams. I was stock serving others and neglecting myself. Many times I sought out to find my dreams, but I could not find them. Then through an awaken moment in a dream, my revelation came true. I could not find the diamond in the sky. I knew that my star had a brilliance, but I could not see it. I once was blind, but now I see. Life has allowed me a second chance to express myself with words. From this moment on I allow myself to mend all the feelings, thoughts, and emotions to create a new version of myself. I had begun to discover my true self. A light had been turn on inside me and I wanted this light to shine from within.

All changes in life require mental adjustment; to release all negative feelings and emotions we pilled up inside to feel secure and protected from the outside world, demands that we completely detach ourselves from them. Our awareness of self-expression and emotions allows us to release, detach, and create a healthy perception about ourself and others. When you become aware of your internal expressions, your thoughts, feelings, and emotions, the outer world is but a reflection of yourself. Transcending from where we are to where we want to be in your life is learning to observe, control, and accept what is without judgments. Only them will you be open to replace the your old image with the new you. It was apparent that my subconscious had kept me blind and unaware of my true gifts. It had play a role in my life to create a minute expression of myself alive-a lie. Undoubtedly enough, I believe everything my mind, my habits, and my thoughts were telling me I was. I wasn't smart enough! I had to depend on others to make me feel important and appreciated. It wasn't until I had my awaken- aha moment that I realized who I am. I am no different than anyone else; I had ideas in my mind that could changed the world, thoughts that where out of this world, and a constant creative imagination. I never stop creating new impressions about how the world could be a better place in my mind. I became interested in reading about Science, Einstein, Dark Energy, The Universe or anything that could spark my imagination. Honestly, I have to confess to you that I became a book worm. Somehow, something had happened, and I wasn't sure of what this was. Because of this creative imagination, I begun to expand my mind beyond my understanding. My mental curiosity lead me to write about science, technology, poetry, with a twist of romance, and my own expressions about the Bible-The Word of God. God only knows what may be next in my creative imagination to write about.

When I begun to write this book, I was approaching my 60th birthday. I felt healthy, motivated, I was dedicated to work on my mental outlook. My morning routines were fill with yoga, meditation, running, and walking my dog. I had decided to move on with my life as a single woman and create my new 60th life anew. I have always being an energetic spirited woman. For me, age has no barriers. I see it as a challenge to create more wisdom in life. Nonetheless, I have to admit that the transition to make a change was not easy. Still, regardless of the journey I was about to take, I was willing to find out what made me move. I had to develop self-discipline, complete control, confidence and become more mindful about what I thought. But this journey was not achieved without conflict, confrontation and pain. I began to develop self-discipline, complete control, and confidence. I had to break the old habit, and believe me, that was difficult; I had to use my old habits as point of reference to improve my future, not as a guided tool into my future. Letting go of habits is not easy, and it can hurt. You feel the emotional pain, as if you were hurting from an injury except, there is no wound. You feel a whole where there is none, and you feel the emotions. It is important that you go through it, or else you will not heal.

There were days when I felt doubt, I wondered how I was going to start my life at my age. I didn't know how I was going to provide for myself. Many questions came up in my mind. Doubts are poisonous thinking. I then picked myself up, and continue to see the future with a positive view rather than a negative one. I employed a new learning strategy, and I understood that from time to time, my thoughts would creep up on me.

The good news was that I could recognize when this was happening and stop it from penetrating into my conscious thoughts. No more unhealthy thoughts, no more old habits. I had to think rationally and transform from the old to the new without compromising my conscious mind.

From time to time, I would wake up depressed and, without hope and doubts will come and go. I understood, that I had to continue my mental training in order to get control of my life. I had to recognize that when I was happy, I would know and understand the emotion; when I was sad, I had to know that a red light was coming on, and I had to analyze the thought and take it to the next level. This process is what many experts will refer to as: brain training. I trained my brain to alert me when my pattern of thoughts was not healthy and productive for my well-being. I had to understand the reality of my subconscious thoughts and make both aspects of my mind work together. I began to understand the mechanism of my subconscious and conscious minds as they worked together with a motivating purpose: one initiated, and the other followed. That's how it worked, and I got it! I had to learn to transform the emotional conflict between my conscious and subconscious minds to maintain order in my thoughts process, or else, I will loose myself in my old negative pattern of thinking.

Imagine building a tall building from the ground up. Each step you take to build must have a very strong component to create a strong support. But what happens if one of your support in the foundation is broken? And the entire foundation is compromised as it loses control? Then what? Do you start from scratch? This is how life works as well. We need a stable foundation to create perfect balance.

Unity is part of the laws of the universe. All things must be in unity in order to achieve balance. Our thoughts, our minds, and our subconscious are supposed to be in the perfect state to create what we want. You, me and all people have the ability to see what it is that causes our minds to stay in a static habitual state and we can set the course to change our minds and conscious awareness. We need to detach ourselves from the old mind, and create a renew mind with an awareness that can expand to our unlimited potential to use the power of our mind. When we expand our mind beyond our limitations, we can discover all the hidden secrets that lay demand within our conscious mind. This is within our basic mental foundation, but somehow it has been disrupted. There must be order in our conscious mind to regain the balance of the emotional loving, caring beings that we are, just like there is order in the universe with all things that exist.

We must be mentally and emotionally well balanced to have a healthy well-being. My analogy here is that as we are, so is everything around us. When we are happy, we seek happier environment, people, and connections. When we are sad, we separate from people and all things emotionally: we disconnect from reality. But when we connect, we seek energy, vibration, power, and all things that are beautiful. When we are balanced emotionally, physically, and mentally with everything in the universe, we expand our knowledge, our spirituality, our belief and our internal and external emotional well-being. Our abilities to love and be loved grows when we are at one with all things.

To connect with all things in this universe, our emotional balance must be in complete harmony with who we are, our happiness, success, ideas, intellect, spiritual being, character, everything we are physically, emotionally and spiritually.

Once you maintain a steady composure in your life, your personal growth and changes happen without conflict or struggles, and you start feeling emotionally balanced in your life. If you are lacking in any of these, you need to work on reprogramming your mind, tapping into your subconscious, and changing old habitual thoughts. Know that your reactive mind is the cause of your mental emotional unbalance. The more you understand your emotional balance and your mind, the better you will be at using your mind to work for you instead of against you. Emotional balance means that you can work with any and all conditions presented to you without a breaking point. When you are emotionally balanced, nothing can take you of balance. Your mind has been trained to connect all the dots before making a coherent thought or decision. Your thoughts are now on higher alert as you take control of your mind. You take control of the situation, not the other way around. You have to master the ability to use your emotions to balance rather than them throwing you off balance in any given situation. Compare this to you driving on a highway , then suddenly, someone cuts you off. You can either get angry or use your intuition to save your life. Which one will you choose? Our minds work similarly, we have to think before we act, or else, we loose our ability to be aware of our actions. When you are self-conscious and aware of your mind, you go beyond the norm. We are used to acting as usual, but awareness requires us to be present, conscious and to pay attention to our actions.

Before I started to write this book, I was writing a memoir about my life. One night I had a dream, but before that I had asked my father in a meditation interval to help me with my thoughts and ideas. I had lost my father three months earlier. In this dream, I had a revelation. A voice in my dream told me to write about my learning experiences rather than talk about my painful experiences. I changed the format of my book and finished it, but before I did, another idea popped into my mind about the power of our thoughts, the ability of our mind to process thoughts, and why. That is how I started this journey to this book.

Before embarking on this writing journey, I was in constant battle with my mind, and my dreams. I was constantly asking myself how and what would I do with my life at the age of sixty. I understood that worrying about my future was normal, but when you have been a housewife with full responsibilities of taking care of everything needed in the house, unless you are stranded financially, you do not worry about this. Moreover, I did enjoy been a wife and taking care of my husband. I took pride in that. What I didn't know is how much my role as a housewife would affect now that I was a single older woman. I had no training or career to help me move forward; furthermore, any interest I had was more of a self-expression than a job. I am an artist creator. I know how to express myself with words, this is what moves me. Plus, I knew I had a very curious mind. I always wanted to know more about the things which interested me; however, at the age of sixty, I had no clue how this would help me build my future. In all sincerity, I felt stock! For the next seven years, I struggled to stay in any job. I had very high expectations from other people that could not be met, but very poor judgment about myself. In my world, people still had common descend and respect; unfortunately, in the new world I was facing, many people values and moral ethics had changed. I wasn't sure I could cope nor adapt to a brand new world. Or perhaps, it was the fact that I was getting older and saw everything from a very narrow view of the world. Having had all the luxury at my disposal for the past twelve years had created a different image of the real world in me. My expectations where but a false assumption of my view at reality. It was here where I begun to do some very deep study about myself, my views at the world, and my lack of conscious awareness about others. And that would transform my life as well as the lives of others. I felt as if the need to manifest my purpose in life had not been accomplished at sixty years of age. Too late? Not according to my beliefs. I had to change myself, my views about the world and of others. Everything I once knew in life had changed, and now, I was but the new older lady around the block. So of speak. Like it or not, I was required to deal with the truth about what had transcended during my twelve years I lived abroad, and create a brand new persona in me. This is how I learned to understand why the subconscious mind refuses changes; undoubtedly, I had become the subject of such an experiment. That is why our experiences cannot be improvise, we learn as we go throughout them, thus become more aware of ourselves. We cannot change what is but rather adapt to it as is.

Lack of awareness is like walking on a river of ice hoping that it would never melt so you don't fall into the deep end. It was my ignorance and arrogance on my part to think that I could have walk throughout my life without having to confront my past painful emotions. For many years, I tried to hide my painful feelings,I acted as if, everything was okay when in fact, inside of me something was crying and hurting. Thus, no matter the efforts, my feelings eventually cut up with me. There came a time when I cry and scream so loud for God to hear my crying, I doubt if He ever did. I felt so lost inside of me. I will cry until I almost lost my voice of past out. Then, I would fall to sleep exhausted from crying. I knew that I had held those tears inside me silently for too long, but I could not suppressed them any longer. I had to let go of my ego. I was in too much pain emotionally to hold on to my sadness any longer. This was the beginning of my transformation. Despite the pain, the disappointment of my divorced, and the loss of my father, I knew I had to deal with those memories and the painful emotions. I had finally released and let go of my painful memories. Now, it was time for me to work on myself.

I understood that I had a path to follow. This was my agenda, or God's will in my life. I had a purpose in my life, and its journey had just begun. You can think big things, but your mind will always find a way to fight your thoughts with the old, negative thoughts. For a long time, I saw things very positively. I moved on with my life and developed a very strong shield. I dealt with my life in the most prudent and logical way I thought possible. My perspective in life was healthy and positive. Although, I had engaged into relationships that were harmful to me physically and mentally, my healing process had kick in. When in the past anger, resentment didn't contribute to my well-being, today, I have learned to remain silence. In that silence, I discovered the deep meaning and power of my mind. You see, before this I would let my family, friends, or husband push my bottoms; but today, I am armed with my mental armer, my self-aware conscious mind. Had I known the powerful influence this silence had in me,

I would have used it as a weapon to restore my mind. There is true value in the power of the mind. As they say" Silence is Golden". My father used to say, "The one who is silence allowed". In other words, silence allowed us to recapitulate and think before acting, doing or reacting too quickly.

I dreamed big, and I had many ambitions. I loved to picture myself in places I had never been to. I saw myself big! I had dreams that were beyond the beliefs of those around me or my deepest imagination.

I believed, that one day I was going to be a big celebrity, an actress, a singer, but never a writer. I did not think that my grammar would help me reach that plateau in life. Little did I know, that one day, I would embark on the journey of writing about my life, science, and technology. I would have never imagined myself expressing words of self-help. My ambitions were of art, design and modeling, but writing never occur to me. This is a good example of how life can surprise you. How life can sometimes surprised us?

Life is full of surprises, and what we see is not always what we have imagined in our lives. I had imagined myself with many children, but I have none; I wanted a big house, and to travel the world, and I did! But I never imagine myself been dependent on anyone else. Just myself. I always had a sense of freedom and self-gratification to know that I took care of myself. I had pride to know I put myself through college. But life changed all that for me. I got married and traveled to places where I experienced cultures I did not know.

I have recognized that life can turn out to be unexpected, but the honest truth is that I had subconsciously planned this life. When I was a child back in Dominican Republic, I dreamed of traveling to America, Europe, and marrying an

American man. Not a Hispanic. Why? I don't know. I had made a choice based on my imaginary projection as a child.

I can honestly confess to you, my reader that I wrote a letter to God asking precisely what kind of man I wanted in my life, and he granted me my wishes, my desires. I supposed you are saying by now, not too bad. Lucky you. But I am here to tell you that you can do this to. This experience of my life had taught me that it is possible to create your future with your imagination. Yes, you can! I did it, and so can you.

Even though our perspective of our lives can turn out to be different, we can change the—path of our future by simply we can tap into our innermost desires then visualize them with our mind. In other words, it is possible to project the life you want, visualize it, and allow the laws of the universe and your beliefs to make things happen the way you want them to be. The key here is no expectations. Do not have any high expectations of your needs and wants; if you do, they will not happen. If you let go and allow them to come to you, the results are miraculous.

When in the past I allowed my unconscious mind and my unhealthy habits get the beat of me, today, I have learned to give in and give it a go. Thus, the results are not always favorable, I know that I have tried my best by forgiving myself and others for any wrong doing. I have learnt that if I care for me as much as I care for others, all is well. I don't have to try to be perfect nor pursue others if they desire not to do so. I am happy with I, the person, I, the spirit, and I the soul. That's where it counts the most.

Changing the world is not our duty; moreover hoping that others change so we can be happy is wrong. It seemed as if relationships brought chaos into my life, or I was simply not ready to deal with the demands of their negative effects in my life. For over the past fifteen years before I got married, I avoid conflicts or confrontation with people or relationships. I kept to myself. I felt safe, secure, but lonely. As result of my getting used to my isolation, I often sabotage my relationships with friends, families or a partner. I had developed a safety net to protect me against the outside world, my loneliness. I then joined a church to help me become more sociable, but that only lasted one year. I felt worst going in than coming out! This is when my journey to spirituality began. I found God in the most lonely and isolated moments of my life, and I felt protected. I was missing nothing. However, my firmed beliefs, created many enemies outside my spiritual protected world. I was constantly harass, and even once physically assaulted by a church member. This would be the last time I would ever visit a church. It has been more than twenty years, and I have yet to step my food into any church. I don't think I ever will again.

I have learned today that this is how the mind plays with our thoughts. We see and perceive life in our own world, not the world of reality. Our brain is like a computer, It processes thousands of thoughts daily. If we allow it to rewind our thoughts, they will continue to multiply as we create more vibration with our minds.

Our perspective in life has lot to do with how we deal with situations, our decisions, and our circumstances. The good news is that life is a continual learning process. Each step gives us and opportunity to improve and lean more about our past and our present, indicating how to redeem a better future. The key here is to be aware when changes happen and to notice how thoughts influence everything around us. Once we change our perspective in life, our dreams become more creative with purpose and fulfillment. Our dreams become more creative, and we find purpose and fulfillment. What matters now is that you have the power to control and redirect your life. From now on, your perspective of the world, and people are the best contributor to positive changes and outlooks in your life and the lives of others. You have awareness and a new aim, in which you see the world with a more powerful view. You can manage and direct your future in the way you want it to go. From now on, the most powerful tool in your mind is your awareness of your thoughts.

I have like to say that our perception of things is but our interpretation about what we see as an observer. Things can be different or change when we are not around nor looking at it. Accordingly, it is a fact that we interpret things depending on our view of what we understand it to be. Therefore, our perception is our interpretation of what is before us, around us or above us, simply put, what we can see or feel with our senses. It is also possible to interpret perception of anything based upon our awareness of their existence, or how they evolve before us. There are many variables to try to fully understand what each individual sees and understand from one single object or subject. Can our perception of reality about anything affect our behavior, our habits or how we process information based on our opinions? Yes, it is possible. This is where the saying "Never Judge a Book by its Cover" comes from. You never know what surprises awaits you on the inside.

Our perception about life, in general, can give us the opportunity to use the most candid aspect of our rational thinking process and come up on the winning side. How we view our internal and external world does affect our behavior, and how we interpret the world. When seeing the world from a narrow perspective, we obscure our awareness of all that is available for us to see. For example, if we make a judgment on a person we see on the streets behaving a certain way, we do not know the reasons for their behavior, all we know is what we see. This person could be an alcoholic, a drug addict, a mentally disturb individual, but we tend to assumed what we don't know by mere observation.

Don't complicate your life with infinite questions, rather, create the answers with the awareness and power of your mind, your thoughts and your energy. The frequency and energy of your thoughts increases all possible outcomes in your life. Just like self-consciousness and self-awareness keeps you mind a tuned, so does the power of your thoughts. That is why projecting a better outcome has to do with you, not the view nor efforts of others. This is how we learn to expand the mind to a higher frequency, with better projections and a more powerful resistance to all negative outcome. All the power is in you! This magnificent intelligent dance between the mind and the brain gives us the ability to think outside the box, create our world, and understand ourselves better. Thereafter, we create a better world for all of us. The more self-conscious we become, the better we are at creating a future with our thoughts. Use conscious awareness to be present, uplift your spiritual well-being and create harmony with yourself and others. Nothing is more tantalizing than to see things evolve before your eyes because you thought about it. This magic is not only available to magicians; you too can do this with your mind. However, awareness of self is important. I have had so many different experiences with my mind that it will blow your perception about what is real and what is not. We are powerful human beings with an incredible capacity to change, transform, create, invent, and make a world of difference.

As we transform how we think, we know and recognize a good thought from a bad one. But how do we deal with this? Can we always think good thoughts? If we did, we could never differentiate between the two. We all know when we do wrong. Just like an animal steals a piece of meat or a child does something he or she knows is wrong, subconsciously they know.

To stay on top of our mindful games, we have to build trust in ourselves. Accept what is wrong, and to recognize what is right. These two opponents cannot exist without the other. Hence the beginning of time, consciousness was created in our logic to help us recognize the difference between the two. When Adam ate the apple from the hands of Eve, he knew not that he was naked, nor did she. However, when they acknowledge their bodies, they became aware of it. This is how consciousness started. Consciousness is an acknowledgment of what is because we are aware of its existence before us. Likewise, you know that a bad or unpleasant thought is an emotional response that brings you down, and feels uncomfortable. To create a balance, you first have to recognize their differences. Understand the nature of your thoughts, recognize where they came from, what brought them about, master your mind, and reject them if they do not serve you. Recognize what is most important to you, become silence for a moment to understand what is going on through your mind; then become consciously aware of what just happened. Eventually, you will learn to master your mind without much struggle.

When you practice mental endurance and mind control with breathing, you can deal with unpleasant feelings, thoughts and emotions more efficiently. It takes practice to quite the mind and control how we think because we have been taught to embrace monkey mind.

If you want to redirect your thoughts, change the way you think by choosing your thoughts. Choose thoughts that give you a better feeling; surround yourself with positive people and positive learning. From the one above. As you continue to implement new strategies to improve how you think. You will create new habits to help balance how you control your thought process. Then you will understand why you think the way you did.

The more you practice at changing your habits, the less resistance you have to confront any situation or conflict coming your way. To recognize something, you must first know that it is there. Accept it without judgments and visualize the transformation so that all things will work in your favor. When you release old habits, replace them with new ones; the release alone will empower you, and your heart will be at peace. Enhancing your awareness with positive thinking helps you create well-being and spiritual coherence. Your conscious connects you to your divine power. This divine power helps you grow and expand your mind with ideas, wisdom, creativity, and more love. You can leave behind all the worries of the world to take action where is needed. Conscious awareness creates a new perspective in our life with a new different outlook. When the worries of my mind over-ride my logic, I create a new view of what I invasion my life to be like. This gives me a new energy to motivate me and change my thoughts. Our mind has an incredible influence about how we perceive all possible outcome. Furthermore, when you take action to change how you think, you are more powerful. This power is what we need to transform how we think and transform the mind. Going to college without a plan for a future career is like you being stock in life with uncertainty; you don't know what you want or which way to go. To create a firm concept about what you want of life or from life requires you to be decisive about what you your future plans. When you experience any blocks in your mind, it is a sign that you need to change the old paradigm. Feel your heart talking to you, listen to your inner voice, and make an immediate change to a positive response of your thoughts. Also, continue to seek all kinds of positive resources that will enhance the way you think.

Immediate response is necessary to make sure that you don't fall back into the trap of your subconscious mind. Stop it at once! Feel your heart talking to you, listen to your inner voice, and make an immediate change to a positive response of your thoughts. Also, continue to seek all kinds of positive resources that will enhance the way you think.

The most positive impact your can make in your life is to feed your mind with new positive thoughts. Once you have become aware of your thoughts, it will be like a clock; you know exactly what time it is because you have learned the numbers by heart. Everything you have ever learned was a learning process.

As you begin to change how you think, you would need to stay grounded and confident about yourself. If you allowed the old shutter in your mind to interfere, you can find yourself creating self-doubts and your fears will take over. When any fear arises, learn to control and take over your mind. This will help you build your confidence and stay consciously aware of your thoughts. Fear and doubts are not signs of weakness; they are a call for change.

Because the response of your thoughts requires an instant critical reaction, your conscious mind takes over and, the response is more effective. So far, you have learned that your reaction to your thoughts are the cause of their outcome. To change you must make a decision to transform or else, nothing happens.

Like a train on a track out of control, the conductor either stop, or continues until the train goes out of control down the path. We too have the courage and power to change our minds.

Release the fear, the negativity, the unhealthy thoughts, and the perpetual state of uncertainty as you build confidence to balance your thoughts from the internal to the external, then you are free!

We are all trained to believe that things are the way they are and that we cannot change them. Wrong! We all have a need to be better, to improve ourselves, and to be happier so what is stopping us? We learned from the old teaching and accept what we learned as truth. We do not choose to believe this way; it is taught from others, and we adhere these beliefs as we grow.

We need to make a personal assessment of our thoughts, and reflect on how to change our conditioned minds. With the power of your mind, you can reframe the old paradigms and replace them with new, constructive thoughts.

The fact that you have pick this book tells me that like me, you too are curious to learn about how the mind and our thought process works. How it is possible for you, I or any one to transform the mind from the old habitual way of thinking to a more positive and healthy state of mind. It takes courage to know that you have a problem, and it requires plenty of guts to change your old habits. Know that healing is painful, understand that you are on the way to recovery, and that changing the mind is possible. Transformation of old habits is possible when your are positive about your thoughts, as well as passive and intuitive about your actions. Certainty and faith are the keys to your success. You will change your thoughts so quickly that you will be astonished at the impact this change has on your life, your actions, and your views of life in general. It is as if the act of taking a step forward to make a difference in your life has turned on a switch that will bring transformation in ways you never imagined possible. You have found a light that will never run out of power.

Your minds ability to make confident changes will surprise you. You will not understand how it is possible that you, a person with such a negative and inhibited pattern of thoughts, could make such a drastic change in a short span of time. It will make you wonder, *"Why didn't I know about this before?"* But give yourself all the credit you deserve, because you alone took the time and initiation to get here. You have gone from a child to an adult transformation by going deep within your subconscious mind. All because you have dug deep within your subconscious mind to rediscover your mental power. But that is not all. You get to be very creative. You begin to discover that this person with a small, captive audience of your own imagination has more potential than you could ever imagine.

You will begin to release and receive knowledge you never thought you had. This knowledge was always there, but your captive mind was never aware of the true potential hidden at a conscious level. Enjoy the journey of your new life experience. You have discovered the key to your future success. The important thing to remember is that this is part of who you are. The past struggles were but a step in the experiences to help you make a profound impact upon your life. You are now the proud owner of your conscious and subconscious minds. You will now determine where you want to go with your life, and you can allow yourself to be creative in ways that are more enhancing to you. Your happiness depends on you, not on the will of any external or internal forces.

Now that you are able to use your mind in a more creative way, the sky is the limit. You can create your own world, you can create your future, and you can be as imaginative as possible with your ideas. It takes imagination, creativity and thinking to make things happen. We all possess that power; we all have the ability to make something from nothing. We have the power of our thoughts to do it. It is an incredible, and magical experience to use your minds ability to see beyond the present and to make something no one else has done before. It takes positive, creative thoughts to do what not one has possibly done. All it takes is you to put your thoughts in gear to think different because you believe you are different. If Nikola Tesla, Elon Musk, and Einstein can think and create new ideas to change the world, so can you.

Don't over exaggerate with reality. Don't dream of something that is unrealistic to achieve, because you will be setting yourself up for failure by aiming where you cannot reach. To think that you can become rich overnight is unrealistic. Unrealistic thinking cannot chance the outcome of your life. Before you can even think about achieving your goals, you first have to set your mind in the right direction. You must allow your mind to deal with success or failure whenever it comes. And you most not put yourself on a pedestal: this will certainly set you up for failure. Success and achievement are a state of mind. Without the right conscious state, one cannot climb the ladder of success.

I love the idea that many people think that they can become successful by reading a book that tells them how. Good luck with that! If you want to achieve anything in life, you first have to accept, breathe and believe in positive thinking. Your habits about daily positive thinking will help you achieve all your goals. It is a fact of life and the law of the universe. One cannot achieve success unless the mind is in the right place, the right thinking, and the right reasoning. Just because you desire something and think about it, that does not mean that you will make it happen. You must think about it with the right vibration, a deep positive conviction, and faith that it will happen.

That is the power of the mind. It all begins with one thought, hope, or light, and then life begins once again. When this happens, you build mental power, life seems to make more sense, and you can understand the power of the mind's ability to think. You go from one state to another and you now concentrate and break old patterns of thoughts. You develop a state of mental power and see things differently; life has more meaning to you. One does not need to die or see the light at the end of the tunnel in order to experience the connection that exists within all things. Even though, sometimes these learning experiences can be spiritually gratifying.

Learn to stay above the negative state of mind and cross over to the light of beauty, a light that not only includes you but all those around you. This perspective helps you think positively, generate positive energy and you receive the same. See negative thinking as a new way of generating a positive outcome from it. Perceive every opportunity given to you as a way to gain rather than lose. Make sure you are aware of how you see yourself, how you talk, and how your life influences those around you.

Know that your thinking power has a big influence upon others, not just you. It is important to maintain a conscious as well as a subconscious balanced mind to influence your outlook on life. Being aware means that you commit fully, now in the present to accomplishing what you have started, you do it with faith, and firm believe that you can. Then you change your illusive mind to think more positively, and you use positive affirmation to reinforced what you have learned. You will be more open-minded.

If you want to explore further into the power of your mind, it is important that you be open to all possibilities. Don't try to be perfect: it is okay to make mistakes, because you will learn from them. Release yourself from old, destructive thoughts about yourself and others. Have positive feelings about you and all those whom you meet. The end result will be spiritually transcendental.

Look for something positive every time you meet someone. Seek only the good; focus on what you have, not what you don't have. Commit to accomplishing one or two things in your life, and it will be fulfilling. Make sure you have faith; take action over fear. Remember that not matter where you are, you have made it this far, so give yourself credit for wanting to be different. Understand that you have the power to change your life with positive thinking and positive affirmation in order to help you improve yourself. Go deep inside your illusive mind and seek to transform your thinking. Practice self-help by putting yourself in a silent state of mind with hypnosis. Utilize prayer, and meditation to elevate your inner well-being. Seek within you all that you are and find your mental power. The worst that can happen is that you will feel better about yourself: you will think clearly, interact with people more openly, and make decisions that will help you focus on your future. You will find that this will bring more balance and happiness in your life.

"BECOMING AWARE."

When you understand the power of your thoughts, you will think more positively about yourself and others, and you will develop an inner intuition that can guide you in your life's path. You will be bountiful, joyous, and open to all opportunities. When you take all this in, you will think not only of yourself but of others. You will share your thoughts with others and expect nothing but unconditional acceptance.

With a full understanding of your mind power, you will begin to love yourself abundantly and radiate love to all with whom you come in constant.

Awareness of your thoughts can expand your horizons to an abundance of possibilities that you could not otherwise achieve. Your positive emotions will keep you balanced spiritually, physically, and mentally. A positive outlook on life and a sense of well-being is how you change your life from thoughts that are misunderstood to those that are not well absorbed by your healthy mind. The more you release negative thinking, the more your positive vibration around you will bring higher positive projections. You will begin to manifest a higher level of consciousness that will integrate with all areas of your life. You begin to align with all your capacities, and will project energy to and from everyone around. You will become the master of your mind's ability to control all outcomes.

Your personality will radiate and glow. People will begin to notice you more, and you will become more confident about your life, and your decisions. A light will shine where there was darkness. Your intellectual capacity will develop without much effort, and you will discover talents you never knew you had. Because your state of mind has changed from the oblique to a new you with energy and healing empowerment, you have discovered a new powerful mental awareness.

Now that your life and mind are in order, you can receive all that is being promised to you by the universe. All your hidden potentials will surface and create a totally new persona in you. The old you no longer exists, your transformation and awareness has taken over.

The negative mind that once procrastinated cannot wait for the next task to create new ideas. You will now experience an acceleration in healing, health, and knowledge that will forever change your life. The miracle is that you have made a transformation where you thought there was not hope.

All the elusive thoughts and false beliefs have been replaced with the inner power of your mind. As you stay balanced, you begin to share all your experiences and knowledge with others. You now have healthy mental outlook. As you continue to experience more positive thinking, you will expect nothing but the best. You will enjoy the pleasures of things you could not afford before, and doors will open for you where you thought there were walls. All this happens because you decided to change your thoughts, that is the wonderful power of the mind. We underestimate the powerful nature of our minds because we are trapped inside our own ideology of what our capacities are.

Some people see the world and their enemies as the cause of their failures. They do not understand that the power is in them; all it takes is a step into the right direction, and all things will follow. It did for me, a sixty-year-old woman; so why can't it happen to you? Think, clearly, dare to change the way you think, and see miracles happen in your life. See how your mind will manifest all that you thought to be impossible. Time, place, race, location and situations cannot stop you. If you can see the light the way I have, you will understand why, a woman of my age took the initiative to make a difference. After all, I don't have much longer to live right? Wrong! It is all in your mind. If I could tell you what dreams I have not accomplished and wish to, you would think I was crazy. But I don't. It is my hope for their realization that has kept my mind alive and striving. I aimed to have my dreams become a reality. If you ever think that you cannot do something, you are already placing limitations upon that opportunity to come to you. A thought is all it takes to make anything happen. Your thoughts are your reality. A healthy mind produces healthy thoughts, so stay positive.

Today, I am the master of my mind. I create my own ideas, and I am the sole owner of all that I create and make happen in my life. Whether you call it the law of attraction or something else, I know that it is my new state of mind and the learning experiences that gives me the empowerment to think healthy thoughts and make the best out of my life.

INTUITION AND WISDOM

Let me share something very important. In the past, I used my mind to guide me through everything I did. I traveled on my own, and made my own decisions to improve my life, all with my own mental power of suggestion. I followed my inner guidance. I learned to use my silence within to managed all external outcomes. I found that we all have a unique ability to intuitively guide, direct and lead ourselves. This is a gift you need to learn to recognize individually. When you do, you will find that this magical ability will guide you in all aspects of your life with confidence and security.

My intuition guides me to understand how I have a voice in me that speaks better than I can; this voice tells me to follow the right path, to stop when I have to, and proceed when I should. If you are experiencing confusion with a decision, listen to your inner voice of intuition. Listen to the conscious voice not the unconscious. The voice that speaks first is the conscious; the second voice you hear is your subconscious rational thinking.

If you are feeling confused, find the answer within yourself. Analyze why your thinking is causing you to feel this way. Stop and replace this feelings with more gratifying thoughts.

Sometimes we are not happy, not because we don't listen to our inner voice or intuition but, because we are experiencing unpleasant thoughts, as a result, we create conflict around us. We are not all meant to be doctors, lawyers or coaches. Your passion is that which brings joy, gratification and fulfillment to you. The good thing is that your intuition will let you know; you inner voice will speak to you.

Intuition can alert you when you are in danger, when you have doubt, or when you are feeling unhappy because you are confused or dissatisfied with a decision. Have you ever done something and found out that something inside you was telling you to do otherwise? Well, if you had listened to that voice, you would have made the right choice. Like I said, the first choice, is the right voice speaking to you. It is *always* right. If you listen to your intuition, you will know exactly what to do. Intuition is like an emergency call that will always alert you of something. Intuition is nothing more than your gut feelings talking to your mind and asking it to follow. Your intuition is part of your six senses. It is that high connection between you, your brain, your mind and that gut feelings with the inner guidance of your spirit-soul.

This intuition can help you survive in critical times, and it can help you with critical decisions when you need to. Intuition is just as much part of you as your soul. If you want to know how powerful your mind is, take a moment to remember a time when you had a thought, and someone closed to you had the same thought. We cannot become thoughtless, we will always think. Our brains process information faster than we can put it on paper. Challenges will make you think, but before thoughts, we have to affirm belief in something or someone. These thoughts can sometimes makes us think and react in a certain ways.

You have the power to forget the past and see clarity in the future, but with wisdom, you can learn to tap into the power of your mind. The brain is an incredible network of information that constantly relates new ideas. Wisdom gives you internal light and enables you to know who you really are. True wisdom puts you in touch with your nature. Your mind shapes that which you perceive, and it is capable of unlimited imagination. Imagination is nothing more than an affirmative thought. Thoughts become reality, and, when that happens, there are no subconscious boundaries. Total consciousness triggers like an electrochemical process, and the brain begins to process ideas. These ideas become a reality, and they manifest with awareness in your mind.

Because the brain is made of memories, not all your thoughts become reality: they are suppressed. Memories become your reality when you unleash the power of your unconscious mind. You can do this by making use of your total mind. You become silence, and seek peace within your mind then, all your questions will be answered. This will help you find your creative capacities. You will begin to relate better with topics of interest and things you appreciate the most. This total brain functioning requires a process of training. Training you or anyone can find with meditation. Meditation will help find your divine power, your silence power is golden and so is your mind.

Your potential will manifest, and your awareness of infinite possibilities will transcend into a higher level of your mind. You will experience yourself reaching a level of being that brings you peace, harmony, and clarity. You will connect to a unified infinite field of silence without boundaries. This peace within will give you the power to think and receive new knowledge. You will connect to an ocean of love and peace. With meditation, you will learn to filter your mind and all its thoughts. You, yes, you can create, and delete your thoughts as you wish.

Einstein said: that the best gift you can give yourself is to expand your mind. Open your mind to a world of all possibilities. Ask, "What can I receive from learning? What can I experience from it? The truth is that reality is more than we think it is. When we make an observation or connect to something by thinking, we discover a world completely different than what we think we know. Imagine if you thought an idea, and then as you turn your television on, you see the idea implemented by someone else. The mind works in mysterious ways. The more you try to understand it, the more you learn and the more you connect to the things you don't completely know. Our minds expands as much as the universe does. As I expand my mind to all possibilities, I improve my energy, I create, protect my inner being, release negative thoughts, and radiate with the universe. I appreciate people, and myself, and I am able to open up and receive the good things that come my way. When we expand our minds to the field of possibilities, we manifest a state of mind that is conscious with all our expectations. Expansion creates growth, growth is knowledge and knowledge is wisdom in all things.

We often do not change our mind because of our beliefs. Our thoughts influence our beliefs. We are not our thoughts; we reflect our inner state of mind with our thoughts, and go ahead and dream big. Your mind creates your thoughts, and your thoughts create your reality. You can create what you want out of life, how you want it, and where you want to go with it. If you can dream, you can make it happen. If you discover the power of your conscious mind, then the sky is the limit. Your potentials are within your thoughts. However, your thoughts must be of a pure and honest nature to know what you want. Sometimes, your thoughts deceive your logic, reasoning, and reality. You may think you want something, but you actually want something else, because something rooted deep inside is hidden, something you cannot see or logically understand. If you allow your mind to go beyond the comfort zone, you will discover not only that you have more potentials than you thought, but that you are able to distinguish between what you want and what you need at the moment. No matter the conclusion, the very nature of your deception will lead you to the core of your need. Nothing happens by mistake. We are a constant vibration that needs to spread more energy to conquer power and acquired success. Seek beyond the now, be open-minded, and allow yourself to grow.

You will flow with all the opportunities available to you, and doors will open where you thought there were walls. Your mind power and your intuition will begin a journey into a vast field of possibilities. Life as you know it will never be the same. You, once thought ideas were only part of a dream, but now will partake in the reality of its manifestation in you. When you look beyond the horizon, you are able to see things that were not apparent to you before. Life will seem as if you are in a constant dreaming state, and you are now the achiever. Your feelings of fulfillment will connect to your true self.

Now you can filter knowledge and information that only you are capable of generating. Through your own vision and passion, all things will be available to you be the universe. You have begun to recognize your supreme being and you are connected to all realms of possibilities. Your inner source will guide you, and you will receive all that comes from within the universe manifestation. You can apply what you learn, your progress will impact your life and others. You alone have done it. You have crossed the bridge of improbabilities and reached your true potential. It is with you that all these started.

But before you get here, you had to believe in yourself, in your divine power, and in your inner conscious mind; the mind that connects you to your true self. You honest, pure self. Before you got here, you had a vacuum, and something was missing; now, you are full of hope, with power, and strength. You have expanded your mind to reach the realm of all possibilities. And you understand that this journey you have taken is not just for you. Your gift is to be shared with others. Your sincerity and efforts are what counts. You have now developed a strong inner core, and you are in touch with your reality.

Have you ever wondered how it is possible that we believe we see all things with our eyes? Think about a time when you had a dream and remembered vividly the details with your mind, as if you actually saw it happen. But how is that possible? You were sleeping and your eyes where closed. Did you actually see something even though your eyes were closed, or did your brain actually interpret what you saw? Sometimes our reality can be distorted, but we look for answers to define what is real and what is not. Have you ever thought about something, and then you hear your partner or best friend say the same thing? Do you wonder how this is possible? It happened to me. I wrote a script, the title. then Jot Down a few paragraphs about my idea, only to see it on the movie screen later. On another occasion, while I watched a movie, one of the actors asked a girl to guess the number of the card she picked; I then noticed that we both picked the same card. Coincidence? It's not. When we think, we create a pattern of energy that can vibrate across distances and into others. I believe that we all have the capacity to create ideas, scenarios, and even visions that are real, but we don't have the knowledge of how it happens.

We are conscious human beings. We connect, and relate, and sometimes we are no fully aware of our own capacities. What is good is that with our thoughts, we can touch the reality of our subconscious, and we give our conscious mind the power to see reality for what it is. Our reality is our ability to distinguish between good and evil, but what we see is not always what is there. Once we understand the dynamics of our minds, miraculous things can happen. We can discover networks of communication between our minds, our thoughts, and our brains to enhance our knowledge of communication. Think of global prayer: together, we all connect at some level. Time and chance can happen to all who try consistently. The good thing is that in communication, we have no competition; the winner of the race is not always the quicker or the most intelligent. Rather, winners are those who are at the right place a the right time. When you are in a place of oneness, with your divine spirit, all things are possible. You will get opportunities, and all things will be within your reach.

The truth is that all reality exists and we tend to accept different answer within our logic. The answers have always been there. Your reality is only deceived because you see things from a different perspective than they actually are; you brain, and your mind are receiving images of false interpretations that you previously learned. Your spiritual awareness will help you align with what is and what is not real. You will receive only that which you want to have. Think with a positive mind, think good, healthy thoughts. If you chose happiness, then you will get happiness. If you choose good, then good will come to you. Change happens when you make a decision to become a better person. When you do, you will bring joy, happiness, confidence, fulfillment, and passion in your life.

Reality can be obscured when we use the wrong methods to achieve success. We gamble, we try the "get rich quick" schemes with motivational seminars, and we dream of a richness that is not realistic within the measures or life; but nothing happens! I call this being at the wrong place at the wrong time. When this happens, you lack the necessary ingredients for success; you cannot do it alone. If your mind and your spirit are not in accord with your desires, you will ask, "How come I didn't get rich?" The truth is that the timing must be right. You must be at the right place, and at the right time, then you can watch miracles unfold before your eyes. It is as if you have touched a genie bottle and wished for a miracle to happen. It just happens! Isn't that lovely?

You may be questioning my beliefs by now. But I say, let's go even further into the mind and all its great capacities. Think for one moment about, from where our thoughts originate. How do they get to our mind? You may think that your thoughts come form your brain, think again. Thoughts can be a mystery of the mind, body and soul. They originate from deep within us. The way you think is the way you feel, express, and act, and that is part of your soul. You act in accordance to the reflection of your soul. In other words, how you feel inside is a pure reflection of what comes from inside your soul.

How can we think from our soul? It is due to deep, inner feelings. It is the soul speaking to the spirit, which then relates to the brain neurons and then goes to the mind. It takes a second to think, but this process is very tedious. Do you really think that the brain simply produces the thoughts without further interpretation of their origin? Thoughts are a perfect manifestation of how you are feeling on the inside. Thinking doesn't just happen; it is created within the deep confines of your inner core, soul, and the spirit. Thinking appears to be easy, but it is a complex interpretation between a set of networks working together to produce a thought. Just because we have a mind and a brain that does not mean that we can process information without having an emotional origin. Once you put all your thoughts together, you would wonder, how it is possible that we have the ability to process a thought, generate this thought to its last possible network, and then, come up with a reason for this thought. The core of all your thought processing begins within that which makes you who you are; your soul! You are not just a body, a mind, or a brain functioning; we are more than that. You are a soul. Once the soul dies, you can't think anymore.

If you think impure thoughts, it means that your soul is impure too. If you think about the state of your inner being at a time when you have an unpleasant thought, at what level do you think your soul or spirit is? Not very good, because if you had a pure thought, then this thought would not have been unpleasant. Think about a time when you felt very loving, generous and kind towards someone.

How did that feel? It came from your loving soul, your spirited being. You are now thinking from the soul-conscious level of your inner being; or the reasonable you, the honest you. Pay attention when you are not feeling at your best, and observe how you think, react and see others; it could not be your best. What this tell you is that your thoughts not only originate from deep within the inner core, but they also tell you what is going on deep within your spirited being.

Expand you mind, discover yourself, and reach the stars with your inner core, your mind, your thoughts, or your soul.

To understand and decipher the truth about the nature of our thoughts, you need to go deep within, experience it, and feel it. Know that the very essence of every living cell in our body makes us think the way we do. Then you can understand the nature of the mind. What really matters to you? Do you want to honestly know who you are, and understand why you think the way do you? Then use this book to discover, how you too can find that magic. Learn to release your old ways and expand your mind. Be open to all possibilities, and be part of this wonderful universe, don't separate from it. Live, discover, understand yourself and others, and expand your horizon to some of the most beautiful opportunities available to human beings. If there is one thing I have learned during my life journey, it is that no matter how we see the world, we all have one thing in common that makes us equal: we are united through our souls. We are a unify set of light that permeates throughout the universe without diversity. Connect, learn, and unite with all the things in this universe; learn that you have the capability, the intelligence, and the mind to do whatever you want out of life. Life is not what you imagine it to be; It is much more wonderful than you know. Indulge yourself in the benefits of living a happier life.

As you trust in yourself, you will learn to expand in this wonderful world. Believe with faith that you can connect to all in the universe, and you will generate the best energy to attract good things to come your way. Believe that you can, and you will! Allow yourself to be open to all opportunities. Learn how your mind and your thoughts are the door to your reality. As you think, so does your soul reflect to the entire world; your mind generates that which you perceive to be you. If you open your heart to see beyond the now, then you will experience a new world of joy. You will learn to open doors to this universe that will transform the way you think for the rest of your life.

The universe is a vault full of treasures and you have the key to it. Open up your mind and find the treasures that the universe has in store for you. If you don't, your life will feel like you are standing still, and nothing around you will seem to progress. Your life will not make complete sense to you. Learn how it can with the three dynamics of your mind, your body and your soul.

Chapter 6

The Three Dynamics of Wisdom

THE MIND

TAMING THE MIND IS A process. The mind has been programmed from a very early age and now, if you want to change the dynamics of why you think as you do, you have to understand the mind, this mechanical tool that does what you tell it to do, wants to control your thinking. Think of the mind as your mechanical tool. Your mind has the ability to absorb information, process it, and then related it to you. The best way to control it is with your energy. Your energy level has to be just perfect, not too high, not too low. This is what I call conscious and common-sense energy. Life in general is about the balance of using your mind power, and understanding how to deal with life in the most rational way. Our mind teaches us how to think for ourselves but also, how to use common sense. When we begin to understand why we think that we do, we approach every situation with more compassion. Because our thoughts reveal how our spirited being is been expressed, our internal emotions are been send out into the world.

If your mind Is capable of processing any information, it is also capable of using a new dynamic to transform itself. The soul dynamic can also be used to change the way you think and come up with a miraculous way to improve yourself. Your mind is connected to your soul, and it has the power to enhance or paralyze your body or your life. When you use your divine power to think, you not only improve the quality of your mind, you also make more conscientious decisions and think rationally. In the end, a healthy and passive way to approach any situation is the only answer. The rational mind is a trusting mind, that thinks before any mental reaction takes place; this mind relates to the soul as well as the body when you think. This mind will not only empower you, but it will empower the people around you. You will shine, and others will see it. The trusting mind does not take revenge, instead, it learns from past mistakes to improve your future. This mind is complete trust, because honesty cannot be demanded.

THE BODY AND THE MIND

The subconscious mind uses the negative energy from the pain of your body because the mind sends low vibrations to your muscles. It relates messages to your mind that are not positive or healthy to your well-being. The keyword here is *well-being,* you the soul, and spirit, are all related. This contradiction of the subconscious mind affects the cells in your body, which then sends negative signals to the body and can produce cancer. The best way to combat this toxic mind is to work on finding a solution to the toxic reaction of the mind. If you try to elicit the best quality of your mind, then you will find it. The truth about life is that we are not attached to anyone or anything in life; we can, at any moment, detach ourselves any situation or thing. You have to think, "*What is the quality of energy I see? When I react with the mind of ego, and I do not experience respect, and the mind of expectations, controls and demands from me.*".

With too many expectations, you will fail, but when you allow your mind to transform gradually, you have no resistance, and will empower yourself. You will use your soul to approach the situation with trust, patience, and you will not fight. Allow things to evolve and learn from them. Your mind does not control you, you control it, its outcome, its thoughts, and its reactions. Say you scheduled a flight, and for some reason, you missed the flight; then you adjust to the outcome by taking the proper action to get on the next flight; don't stress, don't overreact, and don't build-up what is not there. You should cope. You cannot change what has already happened, you can adjust the outcome from here on out.

Your state of mind can subconsciously disrupt the results of your everyday life; and affect your health but only if you surrender to its demands. Take control and, take action in your life's direction. With greatness and simplicity, you will grow stronger. The more you practice, the better you will get, and so will your mind. The mind can make you or brake you. You must find a way to create comfort in your thinking. If you establish a healthy relationship with your mind with positive thinking and good habits, the results will be a healthy body and a healthy mind.

THE SOUL

Physicists tell us that the universe started with a small dot that burst into a space and then all stars and planets began to form. Then shortly after, light began, and we were created. So we are part of every step of the universe's existence. We are a light that was created by the burst of energy that came out of a supernova. We are a soul, we are light, and we radiate here in the universe the same way the stars in the sky do. If we are a soul, a light and a particle of the beginning of the universe, then what makes us tick? What drives humanity? Is it inertia, which is a form of energy. But we are also light, energy, and mass. Mass because we are part of the invisible particles we cannot see but that are present in us and all around us. If we are made of energy, then we are part of the knowledge and everything that is in this universe.

How do you identify who you are: Your emotions, or your physical body? There is more to life than just your emotions and your body. You have to arise from the level of present thinking transcend to a higher level of the self. You are not your mind, but you are what vibrates inside your soul.

The soul is where thoughts arise and subside. Only when you are in a state of consciousness can you understand yourself. Otherwise, you will continue to ask, "Who am I?" We cannot find out who we are if, what is looking does not know how to find it. Every experience is part of an image, a perception, and a sensation of feeling accompanied by a thought. When we can experience the consciousness within the consciousness, we can understand who we are. It is the power of conscious silence; then the internal dialogue inside of us will cease. To truly understand who you are, you must go deep inside your inner core and remain silence. You will find rest and permanence to help you reach the inner you. With your awareness, your mind, body, and your soul will all be in harmony. Learn to use the essence of your soul in you and, act with the forces of your Devine power.

The only thing that matters in your life is the essence of who you are, the oneness. The oneness is the essence, which embraces every living thing. You are energy, the source, oneness, and divinity. The "I am" is the soul. You are not a body, a mind or a thought. You are much more than that. When you start thinking with your inner core, you will no longer use your ego to act. You will see things differently than you are accustomed because, you have made a soul to soul connection, which will take you into a journey to experience a world of peace, joy happiness, unity and a perfectly balance mind. You will achieve a level of consciousness that will help you see impossibilities as an opportunity for new a challenge. Remember that who you are is part of the universe. You are part of the biggest plan that was ever manifested by the creator of this universe, the mind of god, the mind of the "I am." "I am," means you are one with all, you are part of the plan. As you think, so you are. As the great French Philosopher, Rene Descartes Said, I think, therefore, I am.

Now you can embrace your life and flow with the energy and power given to you by spirit of the divine. You are a soul with an eternal brilliance of light that never dies.

When you look up into the skies, know that you, are part of all that was created in that magnificent universe. You are stardust and part of the particles that makes up all of it. Atoms, carbons, oxygen, they all came from a star. They originated from a powerful force of energy.

This knowledge of the "I am" will give you wisdom, and will give you the power to understand why you are here and where you come from. You now possesses the power of knowledge to follow your soul with wisdom. God says, "You are now like me; you have knowledge." The new mind will begin to recognize the power of consciousness hence, you have condition your mind to receive thoughts of pure nature.

You will have only positive thoughts and you will increase your alertness in power, strength, and grace. When you connect with your soul, you are able to see and learn things of magical nature, which will impact your life with brilliance.

By now, you have obtained wisdom and things will become effortless. Good things will come to you without you trying. You will surrender your power to him, and by doing so you will achieve perfect peace. You will know that not matter what, all is well.

Hence you have conditioned your mind not to battle with outside negative energies, you have made a the mental transformation that can only be fulfilled with a higher state of well-being coming from the soul. You have mastered and preprogrammed your subconscious state to respond only when you want. You will unlock a world of miraculous possibilities by controlling your emotional energy source thus, making everything work in your favor. From now on, you can look at your life with optimism and purpose. All the trials in the world could not have gotten you to this point unless you made the decision to be different. People cannot impact the lives of others unless they are willing to take a step forward on their own. With your mind power, you will discover the power hidden beneath your unconscious mind. You have connected the soul, mind, consciousness and total awareness within you. You have discover the source of your being, the soul. Celebrate your transformation!

Celebrate life and know that nothing truly exists unless you are looking for it. Do not worry; if you started it, then God will finish it for you. You are in great hands, you are oneness. The "I am."

WISDOM

As we achieve wisdom through our knowledge from the unconscious to the conscious mind, we develop a well balanced mind and a more rationally thinking mind. Our thoughts connect through our soul because now we are thinking from the core of who we are, not from the subconscious or unconscious mind. We develop a new field of energy from wisdom. Our conscious mind give us the value to deal with any circumstances or people. You consciously connect with your higher self and discover a sense of peace, knowledge, power and wisdom to handle all. This wisdom is power within you and a greater knowledge given by grace. In wisdom, we fill completely satisfy inside, and nothing in us is missing. Spirituality is a quest for unity with the divine through the soul within boundaries of our own efforts. God is not in our brain. The brain processes information via the energy of the soul directed to the neurons and the cells in the brain. God is in our souls, our spirits. God is wisdom. With wisdom you do not look for things to satisfy you rather, you seek the opportunity to share your true knowledge and gifts with others. Success is not the results of hard work or wealth, but the intention to make a difference in you and others. Success cannot be gratifying unless you share what you have learned with others. That is wisdom. To have wisdom, you have to first offer your wisdom to others. A teacher who distinguishes among his pupils, does not posses enough wisdom to teach. You have wisdom when you make no distinction between you and the less fortunate. In wisdom you most first give before you receive.

Give and receive. Wisdom is learned when we surrender ourselves without resistance. We allow ourselves to learn and receive this humbleness, good common sense and compassion. With wisdom, you can influence others, and achieve all things, simply because you have mastered the inner power to achieve greater spiritual fulfillment and knowledge. When you have wisdom, you are patience, kind, loving, and compassionate to others. To have wisdom is to be positive, discipline, and be self-acceptance and acceptance of others as they are. Wisdom is the expression of love reflected from you to all things in life.

As you expand your mind into new horizons, you understand the magical power of positive thinking, and your mind power. It all begins with a thought, which becomes something, it literally creates itself. All human beings have the gift of energy. Our bodies are made of pure energy. We are made of atoms. "We are energy" created from subatomic particles-electrons, protons, neutrons, and more. Subatomic particles are made from energy. We are energy, and therefore we have a built-in capacity to create anything we want. With energy, we expand our minds. The mind is but a creative field of energy. With your thoughts you create power, and this power is the origin of everything you project into the world.

Chapter 7

CHALLENGES ARE GOOD
FOR YOUR MIND

C HALLENGE YOURSELF AND EXPAND YOUR mind. If you challenge yourself with anything in life, you will grow, experience things you didn't know were possible. For me, one of my challenges is to finish what I have started. But I found that in order for me to finish, I must have an interest, or else I will lose momentum. Every time I start one of my writings scripts, or research projects, I always finish it. I can tell you that there is a feeling of fulfillment and accomplishment that comes with completion. I have noticed that when I try to get it done, I am surprised at the end results. When you challenge your mind to do something you enjoy, you will find that your gifts are better than you thought. You will have a more positive outlook the next time you try it. I know from experience that it is not always easy to finish, but that is what makes it challenging. Challenges are good, so keep trying until you get it.

Everything is challenging in life, from taking a new job to moving into a new country, to accepting death as a reality. Life teaches us how to cope, how to accept, and how to prepare for our next challenges. I have had my share of challenges. For example, writing this book was a challenge for me. I had made a promise to myself to finish it. But at the same time, I face the challenge of learning and growing while writing it. Sometimes, growing is painful. We have to accept, learn, understand, and then to put it into practice. Letting go of negative thoughts is not easy, but if we do so, we quickly reset our minds back to our natural balance. When you change, everything around you changes. As Wayne Dyer said. Remember that your brain has been trained to give energy to negative thoughts. When you become aware of your negative thinking, your response to it will be more control, and more objective. Then your brain will automatically respond to your feelings and emotions as you reject negative thoughts.

My advice here is for you to do your best at reshaping your mind and your life. You will find out that peace and joy will abide in you the minute you make a decision to reshape your thinking. It will be like turning the light up in your brain. Just keep trying, the worst that can happen is that you will continue to improve and change. You can now tell your mind to stop! and begin to remember these negative thoughts are not real. Next, you write down how many negative thoughts you have per day and replace them with positive thoughts. The transformation will be remarkable! We all have a more stronger will than we realize. Try it!

I have always said that in order for anyone to be successful and to have money, one first must be happy. The process is changes, happiness, and then wealth. The universe was created as a spiritual training ground for our souls and the purpose of thinking is to put ourselves in control of what we do, think, and say. When I change my subconscious thinking, I awaken my power within. Awaken the giant power of your own mind. If you do, you will be successful, and will enjoy life, even when life throws a punch at you.

Wouldn't it be nice if you took the opportunity to challenge something you love, and you found out that this simple thought brought you a passion you had not discovered until now? wouldn't it be nice if you made money while learning and experiencing what you love to do? Wouldn't it be nice if you could travel the world while doing this passion of yours and share your dream of discovering this passion with others? Wouldn't it be nice if you learned all that from my book? Be thankful for who you are, find your dream, and discover your true happiness with the power of your mind and your thoughts. Challenge yourself in life to find your gift. We all have a divine power within us to do anything we wish. If you discover that power in you, then you will see miracles happen. This power to think, act, and make things happen is given to us by the divine, we simply have to find it. Life is a challenge, and if you take the time to find, and enjoy the many opportunities available to you, then there is a real possibility that you will find happiness, and discover your true power.

It is a challenge to work out, pushing yourself to the limits not knowing the outcome. Sometimes, you can't walk, you feel tired, and your body ache, but you keep trying. You will notice that you can reach further than you thought you could. It its good to set goals and to always do your best. Always follow through; never give up. Even if it means a few pushes, then build on from there. Giving up is not an option.

Another challenge is to pick a topic of interest, whether it is science, physics or technology, and then learn as much as you can until you know it, understand it, and make your own conclusions. I find this challenging for the mind. It is good practice, and will keep your mind sharp, making you think. I find that searching, and learning is very rewarding, if you do it with passion.

If you have any desire for adventure or want to challenge yourself, then follow your heart and do what you like. For me, after I graduated from college, I joint an airline and thus began my first journey into new cultures, new places, and extensive traveling. I flew all over: Florida, Puerto Rico, the Cayman Islands, Nassau, the Bahamas, Jamaica, and Martinique. I went on to Frances, Italy, Greece, and Israel. I love to travel, and it was a great challenge for me to be in new places. I loved the experience of going places I had never been before. I worked and travelled for eleven years before I met my husband, who asked me if I liked to travel.

We got married, and a new journey began. We went to the Dominican Republic and lived there for one year. Then we moved to Nigeria. Three years later, we were in Dubai, and then it was on to Muscat, Oman. After the financial meltdown, we went back to the United States, and resided in Oklahoma for about a year and a half. Then we went back to Dubai which is our current home. If adventure was one of my desires, adventure is what I got!

I need something to keep me busy and alert, and by God, I found it." There were times when I felt like a gypsy: It was pack and go every three years. The challenges and experiences have been panoramic and cultural at the same time. I love the idea of getting on a plane or a cruise ship to go to new places. This is one the many challenging experiences which I always look forward.

My adventure challenges began when I worked as a flight attendant, but I believe the journey is not over yet. This is how the law of attraction works; you wish, plan, and it will happen. I didn't' need to read books to find out. I had learned at a very early age how to attract what I wanted with my mind. I have a gift of knowing what I want and making it happen. How? I think of what I want, I concentrate, I project, and I make the effort and take the first step to get it. Then it manifests into my life. This is how the mind works. That is the reason why I am asking you to use your mind, expand your ability to think, and project what you want in your life. It can happen!

I knew that I love challenges and new adventures. One day I came home to my mother's house and told her I was going to California. California? she said. Yes. I am tired of Florida There are no jobs, so I am going to see what else is out there. She told me, I would not make it, adding, "You will be back." She thought that my upbringing will keep me home, but she was wrong. What she didn't know is that my heart was home, but my passion for adventures was not in Florida. I departed on a journey that would give me independence and new challenges in my life. My independence helped me take life as an expat with ease. Not everyone can live in new places and new cultures, let alone away from home for too long. I have adjusted. I have come to love moving and try new challenges. I have learned to expand my mind and go with the rhythm of life. There were times when I felt homesick; I missed my home and my family. Life is a challenge, and we have to learn to experience in order to grow. If you try new things when you are in a different culture, you might be surprised at what you discover. When I came to Dubai, I wondered what the local people were saying when they spoke Arabic. I wanted to learn, to understand and to connect. I challenged myself to take a class or two. At first I thought, *"There is not the way I am going to learn to write backwards, let alone pronounce this language. I don't understand a word."*

Three months later, I could greet people, and I understood when locals were greeting each other, not too bad for a person who thought she could not speak a word. Then I challenged myself even further and took a second course. I have to admit that my learning skills were put to the test. I could speak it better than I could write it, but nonetheless I learned how to write and read as much as I could. I did my best, and my best was good enough for me. Now, when I sit in cafés and heard locals speaking to each other, I can understand rather than just be ignorant. Is a good feeling. It was another challenge in my life that I was determined to accomplish, and I did it. With challenges comes a feeling of gratification, accomplishment, and fulfillment.

When I was in my late forties, I was faced with the challenge of having too much energy and not knowing what to do with it. One day I challenged myself to run in a thunderstorm with lightning. I remember that only I and another man were at the park. I ran from nine o'clock in the morning until about ten or eleven. It was raining so heavily, and I would extend my arms out to feel the rain on the palms of my hands; it was a feeling of freedom. The thunder was so loud that I feared lighting may hit a tree at the park, and that would be the end of me. But nothing stopped me, and I kept running like a champ. It rained so hard that my shoes were filled with water; I could hear the water inside of them every time I stepped forward. My feet began to hurt. Even though it was raining, I jogged nearly twelve miles without stopping. The feeling was gratifying; I kept on going no matter the pain. I had challenged myself to go with the feeling of freedom and the joy from the rain rather than stopping. Just as I approached my tenth mile, I realized how much rain was on the ground. Once I stopped and went home, I felt numb. I had a feeling of gratification, but not without pain, my feet were on fire, and I had blisters. Even so, I felt a rush for pushing myself as far as I could. Then, I got stuck in traffic for three hours. My car was flooded with water while waiting in the rain. No cars could move there was not place to go. I saw big utility vehicles stuck in water. Today, my energy has not subsided. I still run, ride my bike, walk, do yoga, and palates. I will remain active until my body says I can't anymore. Is my power of determination that keeps me going.

Challenges sometimes can result in tragic endings. I took the advice of a yoga teacher while living in Muscat, Oman, and participated in a cycling class. As I got on the bike without further instructions from the teacher, I got my foot cut on the petal, which further ripped my leg wide open. I could see the bone inside my leg. I couldn't feel the pain, but I froze for a moment, and then the pain started. I had never been in a cycling exercises classes, but I took the challenge to try it. I didn't show any weakness or fear towards it, but I paid the price. I can still see the scar on my leg, but it is now part of the past and is only a story, nothing else.

One summer when I visited Hawaii on a cloudy day, I went up to a waterfall with some friends and sat by the beach. While we were sitting and having a relaxing time, we couldn't help but watch this lady trying to jump from a ten-foot cliff into the water. We watched her try for almost forty minutes without success. She would get to the edge, try to jump, and then move back in fear. I couldn't stand watching her. I told one of my friends to watch for me. I was not a good swimmer, and I knew the water was kind of deep. I walked up to the cliff, looked down once, and then jumped. I had done it! The only bad thing to come out of it was that I bruised my pinkie toe. It was fun. I feel that if you are going to do something, you should just do it or step back. Nothing is ever accomplished with uncertainty. It is good to take challenges within reason. Trying new things can be challenging, so make sure you make wise decisions.

I believe that we know when something feels right and when something does not. Listen to your inner voice and go with it. There have been many times when I heard my inner voice speak to me, but instead I listened to other peoples' opinions and I fail. You must learn to listen to that voice that warns you when you are in danger. We all make decisions based upon how we feel and think, and we must use our judgment. Think wisely. Thinking is the essence of every action we take. There are times when we must remain silent in order to listen to our inner voice. We cannot always find the answers to what we are seeking if we allowed our thoughts to interfere. Sometimes it is important to be quiet, say and think nothing, and go deep within. When you asking for questions, you will find the correct answers because you always knew it. The only thing that was missing was your awareness of your thoughts.

How do you know when to listen to your inner voice? When you are aware of your feelings, your emotions and your thoughts, you are in touch with your conscious self. This conscious self is part of your internal voice of wisdom. It is with this voice that your conscious speaks to your heart. This interval voice tells us when we are in love, happy or in danger.

You will understand this feeling in you and, it will manifest at times when you need to know something. Sometimes, unless we know how to use the gift of listening, we cannot hear the internal voice. You will not know the outcome of anything unless you understand the nature of your inner voice, which will help you survive when you face a real life challenge.

I once heard someone say, "I don't need a book or lessons to teach me how to make decisions or tell me what I want in life." Life is a challenge, and we all need to experience different facets in order to know the truth. How can you know reality when all you know is perfection? Life is neither perfect nor without challenges. To this I will say, blessed are you who know all the answers for, you have nothing to share with the less fortunate.

For me, one of the greatest gifts in life is to be able to share that which I have experienced. Life is what we experience while climbing the mountain of challenges. We cannot share the experience unless we have experienced it ourselves.

Unless Jesus and other prophets experienced what we know today, there wouldn't have been any religion for those who believe. Whether or not you are a believer I leave it up to you. I am not trying to preach; I am simply making a hypothesis.

If you know the true value of life, you will do all that is within your power to challenge yourself and fulfill your desires. You can always discover something new and exciting. Today, even though I am approaching sixty, I do not fear to try to reach new desires or goals. For me, age is only a number, not my reality. Reality stops when you give up your dreams and cease to be who you are meant to be. I believe the best is yet to come, and I still dream big! I know that one day, I will see my script on the movie screen. I know I have the imagination, and I what it takes. Do you want to know how I know that? Because I get that feeling whenever I am watching a movie. There is a gut feeling inside of me that one day I will see my name. I know it, I see my name on the movie screen, and it says, "Frances, Screenwriter." That is me. It all starts with a belief and then everything else follows through. When it happen, I know that this will be a wonderful day for me.

If using my mind is a challenge, I want to keep my mind busy: I like to read and keep my mind busy. It helps me get through the days with a feeling of accomplishment and understanding. I've found that being busy keeps my mind in a healthy state, and my cells and neurons grow. It is funny how things work out in life. My college favorites courses were not physics or science, or math but today I challenge myself to learn all I can in these areas. I was not interested in math, but I can definitely count and keep track of my finances. I had to lean. I had a very difficult experience after a surgery where I lost everything I had. I had to start from nothing and pick up all the pieces. I know how hard life can be. Because I am open-minded and expand beyond the now, I have challenged myself to learn from everything that is available out there. I am thankful for all the information available on the Internet, which can help us grow as we wish. Although challenges may come in different ways, I still consider what I have done a challenge because it took determination to do what I was not willing to do before.

Chapter 8

NOW WHAT?

YOU MAY BE ASKING, I know how to control my thinking habits. Now that you have learned how to use the power of your mind and change your habits and be aware of your conscious mind; don't ignore your subconscious mind power. Follow your dreams, and do not ignore your thoughts. Our thoughts are not something inconsequential; they have power and energy to influence how we think. You know how to express your feelings and emotions; you can remain calm when you have to; you can be aware of yourself as a soul and spirit with self-love.

What you think is part of how you feel. Your thinking is an expression of how you feel, how you project, and how your brain receives information sent from your neurons to your mind. It is all interconnected. Positive thinking evokes shades of light in you and all around you. If you regain your sanity from negative thinking habits to good conscious thoughts, then you will have back your voice of reason. Remember to carefully choose your thoughts to maintain awareness in your thought's patterns. Maintain awareness in your thought pattern. Carefully choose your thoughts.

Your thoughts represent all aspects of your life, internally and externally both. As you go through the day, stop at every moment you have to say something or express your inner feelings. Your thoughts are part of your individual state of mind, as well as what is been recorded in the visual cortex of your brain. Your thoughts are the results of your past preprogrammed state, or the subconscious mind. The more you slow down the process of thinking before speaking, the better you will get at controlling your thoughts. Remember that you are powerless over nothing; if you want to a change, you can. Nothing is impossible if you wish to conquer it! I have found that as long as I put my heart and belief into what I am doing, I will eventually get it. But I must use logical thinking to make my ideas come true. Because your brain helps you process information, you are responsible for bringing your thoughts in order with your mind. Your mind has to be clear and in a perfect order, like a group of thoughts that will complete themselves. Thoughts are like a narrative; once it starts, you can create a story and develop it with a group of related thoughts.

Cells generate new cells which in turn helps your brain generate new thoughts. Nature constantly changes, and so can you. Learning to train our minds to think different is not impossible; all it takes is a new thought. If you are determined to make a difference in the way you process your thoughts, then all it takes is one moment, one thought, one millisecond. As you explore your mind, you will discover that you are not limited by anything; only your thoughts limit you. Your own need to grow will get you there. Don't change so that you can please others, change for yourself. In moments of desperation, turn inward, go silent and find the answer. Maintain your faith and in what you believe to be true. Remember that all journeys require effort and dedication.

You have something to offer to the world and others. Stay conscious in the present and cut out your subconscious mind from your future plans for success. Move into a state of allowing to help you clear your mind, and open your heart for good things to come. Listen to that voice inside you that tells you what is wrong and what is right for you. Do not listen to the voice of doubts in your mind. Always read and pick subjects of good and healthy nature; do not read anything negative that can bring doubt or negative feelings to your heart. Communicate with people who share your dreams and connect to those who are at your spiritual level; they will help you grow. Remember that your brain has at least one hundred million cells that constantly multiply. Thinking and processing good thoughts helps your cells grow, so nurture your brain and create good habits. Thoughts give birth to new thoughts, and what you think becomes you. Think positively, and project a happier and more balanced self. Our knowledge of the universe is constantly changing, new elements, new planets, and the forces of nature. You to can change your thought patterns, and your personality, transforming your life to be better.

Be aware that there is a new awakening going on in society today. Our technology and our ability to gather information today is more prevalent than ever before, and information is at our fingertips. What you can learn and are able to do with your brain is entirely up to you. The amount of data available is insurmountable!

Nothing is impossible anymore; it is all about what you as a person want out of life.

The lessons I have learned in my life, are of my own making. My stubborn way of thinking, and my constant battle with the subconscious mind got me where I am today. My ego got in the way many, many times. But I will make it clear to you: I have no regrets. My learning experiences have created a journey I will never forget. It is with this passion that I can stand by you and tell you how to make a difference in your own life.

No matter what happens in your life, this is not about you rather, it's about how you can help others while getting through this journey in your life. I did, and so can you. I found the strength and I had a light shining over me and guiding me here; I think it has to do with my father, after he passed on. Know this, what your mind thinks, perceive and believe, you can achieve. If you understand this, nothing within your reach will ever be impossible in your life. You can create whatever you dream.

You create your own future, and your own life drama. You are the protagonist of your stage performance. Try sometimes to act out your life drama, your mental outlook will completely improve. Remember that the results of everything in your life are the byproduct of what, how and when you are thinking. When you think positively, the laws of the universe will work to help you project your desires. Your awareness of your thoughts will teach you how to use the power of your thoughts to help you manage through the day. Use gratitude to enhance your life and be thankful for what you have now, even if, you are going through bad times. Be thankful for where you are today, because tomorrow has yet to come. If you wish to move forward, you must first be thankful for what you have. If you do, your life will change. Life is about being positive even in the worst of times. Know that in crucial circumstances of life and death, survival may depend on a positive state of mind. Even if you are unprepared for what happens next, don't look back. Use the past as a guided tool to improve your present and your future. You will know when you have acquired clarity in your way of thinking; you will begin to change, and all things around you will change. If you don't change, you will constantly engage in similar situations asking yourself, why things turn out the way they do. As you begin to change, your life, your knowledge and wisdom will improve.

I am also thankful for learning about different cultures while traveling, for the opportunity of learning about languages, and religious norms. It has been a journey of joy, learning, and nostalgic feelings. Being away from home can make me home sick, but, It is worth it. I wouldn't change it for the world.

I am certain that there is someone out there wishing he or she could have had this opportunity. I am grateful for this moment and I know that my desires made this happen. I wanted this, I wanted to be in different places. I wanted to experience different people, cultures, and places. I trained my brain to bring me what I wanted by thinking about it and making it a reality in my mind. Some may think it is destiny, but I say it is our desires and conscious mind that think about what we visualize, then the moment begins to evolve as a reality. You get what you want. So wish for all you want and more. Don't just think about the moment, think big! The universe is waiting out there to make it happen for you. You know your thoughts can become a reality. Put them out there, and then put it into practice. Go ahead and think big! You will find that you have the power within you to make everything happen in your life if you dare to think it.

With positive thinking and understanding, you will process all things in faith as you belief in yourself. This is not a quick fix process, but it certainly works if you keep trying. I see it as part of nature where, everything is governed by past experiences, a present situation, and a future outcome, but most of all, by your thoughts.

For me, the quest is not just to finish this book, but to continue the search for an idea that will transform the universe, the way we understand science, technology, and the things about our creation we don't understand. I see life as an opportunity to indulge into the many opportunities available out there to make an impact with a new idea. When I finally do, then I will have truly rediscovered myself.

Yes, I am a dreamer, and I place not limitations when it comes to dreaming new possibilities, new ideas, and new creativities. I think that when it comes to ideas and creativity, the sky is the limit. We can dream, manifest and we can make the impossible with our minds. How many great geniuses began with just one thought? It was a thought that change the history of science when Einstein discover the mathematical calculation of E=MC2; or when Galileo made the remarkable discover that the earth orbited around the sun. Thinking is the most powerful influence in the world, with a thought, you can change the world.

You don't have to be a genius, but you can come up with an idea and transform yourself as well as the world around you. You can do anything you can imagine in your mind. Anything!

Stand by your beliefs; don't let anyone talk you out of your creative thinking. Believe in yourself and now the truth. Don't question yourself, just do it! If you fail, you will discover a new way to deal with it and add to your knowledge. The next time you are faced with something similar, you will know exactly what to do. You will analyze your thoughts, improve and transform the way you think. Life requires that we go through a series of transitions in order to learn from it. These transitions empower our thoughts and help us function as conscious human beings. The more we learn about the mind, ourselves and life, the better we are.

Wouldn't it be nice if you came up with an idea that impacted the world? Or if you could discover something that no one else has thought of before? Wouldn't it be nice if you left a legacy that changed the way we think forever? Wouldn't it be nice if you had all the comfort, happiness, you had dreamed to have in your life? Wouldn't it be nice if, I could travel all over the world because you are able to imagine it?

Think and know. You have the power. Write down any ideas you may have and try to develop them as you go. See what you can come up with but before you do, imagine this idea already happening in front of you. Live it, enjoy it, and act as if it has already come to a reality in your life. Picture it, visualize it, and see it happening in front of you; this will help you transform your ideas into reality. Think of the fact that all the building blocks of life came from space. We didn't know that years ago but recently, the persistence and tenacity of a few scientists helped them discover the truth. Carbon 13 was found to have its origin from the solar system. Creative ideas help us shape and understand our true potentials. To think creatively, you must stay mentally positive and visualize everything with a positive outlook because your state of mind is imperative to the outcome of your thoughts. If you are in a good mood and have a good attitude, chances are, you will have more productive thoughts.

If you are waiting for something to happen in your life, but it is not happening, there is a high possibility you're projecting part of the outcome. It is very possible that doubt has come into your mind. Therefore, it is important that you choose your thoughts carefully. Remember one thing; your thoughts are like a magnet, and will attract what you desire. If you think positive thoughts, keep the good vibration in your mind going, send the same to your subconscious mind without one single negative thought. The results will always be more positive. Because your thoughts have a magnetic field, they will attract your feeling inside of you. It is what you feel that attracts your thoughts. Feed your mind with creative and happy thoughts. Always think positive so your thoughts can manifest like a magnet.

As you are thinking, the law of attraction is responding to your thoughts, desires, needs, and wants. But always remember that everything relates to the origin and nature of your thoughts. Your thoughts are like an echo and they send out vibrations into the universe, which then return to your mind at a higher vibration, the higher the frequency of your thoughts, the more magnifying the results.

Ever wonder why you keep thinking about an issue or situation during the day, and you can't seem to let go of it? This is a good example of how the frequency of your thoughts can be magnify. Thoughts, whether they are of passive or aggressive become action. When we express anger, it is a response from our aggressive state of mind or our emotional reaction to a thought. This aggressive nature is what makes people commit crimes. But first, they have to think this aggressive thoughts, and then anger does prevails with deep emotions.

Passive thinking, on the other hand, reflects a calm and loving nature with positive loving thoughts. Contrary to what you may believe, passive thinking leads to passive behavior with candid and compassionate feeling towards others. This is the state of mind you want to embrace in life.

Process what you want with good healthy thinking. If you want positive results in your life, you have to maintain the balance of a positive outlook. Remember to stay positive, and you will attract nothing but the best. Good things come to those who are positive, project healthy thinking and maintain a balanced state of mind.

In 1994, I packed my small Civic Honda and my cat and took a trip to California, Amarillo Texas, Vegas, San Diego, and Finally to Utah, Arizona, ending up in Houston Texas; I knew that I will never look back. I felt something inside of me driving, and moving me forward to experience new places, so I did.

To this day, I have not regrets. It is good to challenge yourself to do things differently from the norm. For me, it was important to go with my inner feelings and follow my path or destiny. This is the reason why I am here today to share my journey with you.

The power of your mind can help you expand your view of the world, and take challenges, that can help you experience new horizons. The mind is a creative field, a field that can be explored as long as we are willing to go further than our comfort zone. Get out of your routine and do something different. Life is a marvelous challenge. "Take a chance." When you experience new cultures, you open the door to new understanding and appreciation of something you didn't know. You will exchange cultures, and leave with a sense of awareness about yourself and others. The good thing is that, experiences, feelings, knowledge and understanding as well as culture will be share. Expand your mind and experience a new world of knowledge.

Because our mind has two states, the conscious and the subconscious. In order to maintain a fresh and healthy outlook, as well as a balanced mind, I take the following things under consideration. I center my beliefs in who I am, as a soul. I know I am not the color of my hair, the color of my skin, my success, or my failures. I accept myself and others for what they are; a soul. But most of all, I think positively, and that is the balance. You can also make a promise to think differently. Here are some examples of promises I've made to myself.

- I will invoke positive intentions with my thoughts about myself and others.
- I will hold my dreams graciously in my daily thoughts.
- I will always surround myself with positive people.
- I will project energy that reflects my love, compassion, joy, and my wisdom.
- I will not take things personally.
- I will make no assumptions about myself or others.
- I will be impeccable with my choice of words.
- I will make my house and my surrounding as comfortable as possible.

As you come to understand the purpose of this journey in my book, let me remind you how to stay constant with your thoughts, your beliefs, and the truth. Remember to stay in the moment. Remain authentic with your thoughts and be guided by your soul. By connecting with who you are, you will think more positively. You will be a better listener and operate from your intuition rather than your subconscious thinking. Know the truth and consciously trust and understand your emotional vibes as you receive them.

What is the truth you may ask? The truth is who we are. We are a soul, and the soul is the only truth there is. A soul is the root, it is God, and it is reality. The truth is the only reality there is; it is the knowledge of God. Being truthful means that you are eternal, that you are honest with yourself. If honesty is not part of who you are, then you cannot embrace the truth about others; that which you don't have, you don't understand. Remember that as you give, so shall you receive. Go inside yourself and find the truth within. You will know that truth is power, knowledge, and self-consciousness. Truth is self-awareness of who you are. Know the truth, and it will set you free. You have to know yourself, in order to understand others. Love yourself, in order to love others. You cannot recognize your brother if you don't know yourself. It is easy to judge without knowing the truth if you knew the truth, you would not judge. Truth is doing something that brings you and others joy. If you do, you will find true happiness inside.

Find something that brings pleasure in your life. The only way to be fulfilled in life is to have goals, positive outlooks, and dreams. Without these, you are just here, and you only exist. You have no purpose. Life is too short, and sometimes happiness comes in intervals, so find joy in what you do, even if that joy is doing something that makes you act like a child. It is the child in you expressing happiness. Waking up with feelings of sadness and despair is not good living. I have been there many times. I experienced this during the loss of my babies and of my father. I could not understand why I was feeling so miserable inside. It was not until I started to write it down that I began to learn about the process of healing. I had to live the experience all over again, and it was painful. I felt as if I had gone back into the past and touched that which I thought was no longer part of my memory. I had to do this in order to know the truth. I had to understand my feelings, my memories, my sadness and my loss. Recording back to these feelings really hurt.

Life is full of choices, but you have to think for yourself. Don't gamble with your decisions. Think for yourself and be positive. For me, making the decision not to be a coach was the right decision. I was happy letting go of something I could not control at the moment; it wasn't the right time for it. That choice brought me here to share my life with you. Sometimes making the right decision can be very rewarding. Don't get stuck and unhappy with your choices. Do what makes you happy.

What wakes you up in the morning? What brings you that feeling of fulfillment and joy everyday? What makes you think and be creative? When you know, you will find your true passion. Believe in yourself, and you will do it. I believe that everything is possible. Sometimes I dream big! and I see myself in places I've never been, acting roles I have never played. My dreams will remain alive until I die, because I believe that all things are possible, even in the illusion of my creative mind. Dreams keep me alive, keep me thinking, and continue to help me create things of an unforeseen nature. I dream without limitations. You can try to be conscious, but you cannot protect yourself from all outcomes all of the times. Allow your life to unfold, but don't be obsessed about making things happen for you. Stay with the right attitude, the right view, and right mindset. Things will come your way. You will feel it when it happens.

It is easy to give in when things don't happen the way you expect, but you have to keep chasing your dreams. Like everything else, if you are persistent, it will eventually pay off. Once you aim for it, never look back. Remember that successful people don't give up easily; they are constantly working with their goals and choices. The word no doesn't exist in the mind of an achiever. Know that you can do anything you want if you are truthful and dedicated to it. Take risks and know that you will make mistakes. You will learn, and your experiences will make you stronger.

This has been an amazing experience, and I have learned many lessons. I learned that to find the solution to my problems, I have to jump into the core of the problem: my mind. I study the mind, the brain, and conscious and subconscious thinking. I found that I have a curiosity in my mind that never stops. I try learning about any problem by digging in and finding the solution for myself. My suggestion is that whatever your dreams are, read about them, study them, and have fun in the process. Don't follow any rules; stay focused and create a habit of dedication to whatever you are doing.

I do things with a tremendous amount of passion and dedication. It has been said that if you want perfection, you will not find it. I believe that unless you are dedicated and passionate about your goals, you will not conquer them. Perfection comes when you make the best of what you love with passion. Your inner fervor and drive inside you will help you make a difference one day. That in itself is your perfection. We are neither perfect nor imperfect; we simply learn by trial and efforts.

I have written scripts for movies that were never published. I wanted the enjoyment of something to do, to fulfill my passion. I have five scripts that have been stacked away in a box for ten years. The greatest satisfaction is that I had fun writing them. I believe that the experience of acting out your passion is worth more than money. In the end, you never know what you may discover, because life is full of surprises. I believe that success comes when you continue to work on your dreams until something comes of it, and you never give up. When you remain true to yourself, you never know what you may find. You may find out that what you have been so passionate about is now your greatest gift. Painting is one of my many passions. I started painting after my first divorce, and; I began to rediscover myself. I am persistent with my dreams, and I do what brings me happiness even if it is not perfect or makes me money. Fulfillment is not about benefits; it is about gratification and self-expression.

Closing Words

WHEN I STARTED TO WRITE this book, I was inundated with many negative thoughts in my mind. But one day while confronting a situation with a coaching course, I decided to take a turn for the better. I decided that I had to put my mind in the right perspective, or else my future would be oblique without a happy ending. As I wrote the book, not only did I learn to accept what was wrong with me, but I began to love my life, my intentions, and my new habits.

Something inside me had changed. I began to live the life I always wanted: a life with purpose and without conflict. This happened because I stepped into the very core of what was causing a constant reaction around. I jumped into my subconscious mind and took back my life. I stopped the constant negative habits that had lived in me for such a long time, and I decided to take charge of my life. Today, I am happy not to have taken the coaching course. I understand that in dealing with my problems, it helps me understand the problems of others.

Sometimes we are unable to see deeply within unless we go to the root of the problem, the truth. I encourage you to take a look deep inside the root of your problems, your thoughts, and your subconscious habits. Dig deep within and transform what is causing you to think the way you do. It takes guts and courage to start, but once you do, you are on your way to a healthy living. Take it from me, because I have been there. Life is a beautiful experience that deserves to be enjoyed with happiness and pleasures. Don't deny yourself the wonderful opportunity to be part of the joy. It is never too late! It took me a long time to get here, but I am happy to be at the right place, and at the right time in order to enjoy this unforgettable experience. It is my heart's desire that you can find comfort in the way you transform your life with your thoughts.

Once again, let me remind you that your conscious and your subconscious minds do play a very important role in how you think and react.

I hope that after reading this book, your life will be blessed with a new positive perspective. This can only happen if you take the initiative to make a change. It all starts with you! If you don't take the first step, your life cannot be blessed and transformed.

I have explained in great detail how to think positive, and how to use the conscious mind instead of the subconscious to help you discover the power of your mind. And how transformation can be a blessing to help you change your life with the truth you will find in this book. If you have been blessed after reading it, I hope that you keep practicing with the powerful foundation of your mental efforts.

This has been a blessing for me, and I enjoyed the journey of your company. I hope that I have given you a gift of love and blessing. Remember who you are: you are a soul, and you are part of all that is in this universe. You are energy. As God is, so are you.

He will cause you to shine in every aspect of your life.

I hope to hear from you about how this book have empowered you to make a change and achieve success in your life.

Till we meet again,

Frances Mahan

About the Author

FRANCES MAHAN PURPOSE IS TO bring clarity to the minds of millions.

She began her journey with a dream, a dream that started years ago. Her destiny insights and, eagerness to do what she was meant to do in life took her further than she ever planned. After losing her father, Frances had a dream that brought her clarity so she could write this book about the power of thoughts, the mind and her spiritual experience. She had to understand her own mind and she discovered that she had the ability to process information with her mind faster than she could put words down on paper. This beautiful journey led her to an enlightenment of compassion and awareness of herself and others.

She learned that the mind and brain are connected not a mystery. Her understanding of the mind was a pure experience while writing this book. She discovered how to regain control of her mind and use its power to be more productive, to connect with her spirited self, and to have a successful life. The end results were, her ability to control her mind and building confidence one day at a time. She listens to her spirited being, which brought light into her life and began a healing process to bring light where there was darkness.

Because she was determined to go through the experiences and mental transformations on her own, she can now share this with you, the reader. While she wrote this book, Frances was still traveling; she was a housewife but was looking for something to satisfy her dreams. She knew that for the next ten years, she did not want to be doing the same thing she had done for years. This is the reason why she embarked into a journey that discover what she really wanted to do with her life. She wanted to experience freedom, and a complete sense of satisfaction of doing something for herself and sharing it with others. She wanted to discover her true self. In the process, Frances experienced immense learning; mental, spiritual, and self-healing while writing this book. This remarkable experience brought her peace, wisdom, and true happiness. For her, writing this book is an experience that let her understand the old habits of her subconscious mind. She used writing as a form of self-healing method to improve her life and understand her mind better. Her writing journey has been an uplifting spiritual experience as well as a healing prophecy.

Because she experienced an amazing growth, she wants to share all her learning experiences with your reader. She learned that the mind has an incredible ability to take information and process it as far as we commanded to; she understands that memories and the subconscious mind can impair us from moving forward, and that we have control of everything we think and process in our mind. She understands that we are what we think, so she is now more aware of her thoughts.

Note from the Publisher on "Lotus of a Conscious Rebirth"

THINKING IS A MIRACULOUS ACT of the mind. To create anything with just a thought is a powerful process of the human mind. Most of us utilize our time thinking about problems or reflecting on the past, rather than focusing on the present. We forget that our capacity to create new ideas is in us, in our minds. The brain has about one hundred billion neurons and these neurons generate energy, which then produces cells to enhance and improve the mind and our thinking. The ancient Greeks wondered why the mind creates and gives meaning to thoughts. Why do we have consciousness and evolve as human beings? The reason is that we have awareness, which creates consciousness. Consciousness leads to understanding, and acceptance of the truth in us.

In my words, I share how my thoughts and my mind kept me from achieving my success and being who I wanted to be: a free-spirited person. I talk about how I overcame the mental blocks with my own willpower. I searched deeply to find the meaning of all that was happening to me without resolution; then finally, one day I had an epiphany, and everything became clear to me. I began to change my mind about the old, and embarked on a new journey of self-healing. This experience led me to write this book, but as I was writing, I began to feel an uplifting spiritual experience. This simply confirms that thoughts can create everything and anything in your life. If you want something to become a reality in your life, all you have to do is projected it, and envision it with your thoughts in your mind, it will happen. I found that I had no limitations: they were only set by my own view of reality

Thoughts have power: they become what you think, and they have an energy that carries what you think as long as you feed it more thoughts. Thoughts can become reality; they have the power to manifest themselves in your life because you give them the power. Understand how the power of your thoughts can make a big impact on your life. Feel the flow of my words as they describe to you what negative thoughts can do and why positive thinking can make anything happen in your life. With your thoughts, you can make your dreams a reality; you can reach further than you thought possible, all because you thought of it. Your thoughts are priceless!

You can overcome any obstacles with your mind, your thinking and your views of life.

Every situation in life brings us an opportunity to express our thoughts in a more positive and productive manner, thus combating the habits of our subconscious mind. Learning to manage our subconscious habits is a reminder to be constantly aware of our thoughts. It is like having unhealthy breakfast to feed your body, except you are feeding your mind with positive healthy thoughts.

When we think positively, it brings good vibrations into our harmonious life, and things evolve with ease. Things fall into the proper pattern of order in our lives and our expectations. Positive thinking is not only good for the mind, and your body but, it also balances your body hormones sending signals to your brain that brings a sense of pleasure or fulfillment.

My hope is that this book helps you understand how to transform your old thinking habits. Improve and excel! I want you to see how it is possible to change the way you think and become a better, healthy, and positive person. Use your thoughts to improve and release the clouds that are stopping you from being positive. Meditate, be aware, and transform your thoughts as you change your life.

I hope that you pick what is best for you and put it to use in your life. It is my intention to take you on this journey with me and lift you up where you have been let down by your mind. It is my deep expression of life that brings me closer to you the reader, and my virtue of sharing all my growth and experiences to connect with you.

May the contents of this book help you find the key to the most powerful energy in your mind, so you can achieve all your desires. Be happier, and live a miraculous life. With love and compassion, I hope that you find encouragement in my words.

This has been a blessing for me, I have enjoyed this mind transformation with a happy ending. My desires are for you to have the same results. I wish you find peace of mind and a new way of looking at life from pain to freedom.

Thank you for reading my book.

Remember that you are loved!